Atopic Dermatitis and Pruritus
Interesting Cases

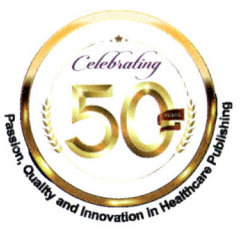

Atopic Dermatitis and Pruritus
Interesting Cases

An initiative of
Atopic Dermatitis Centers of Reference and Excellence (ADCARE)
Global Allergy and Asthma European Network (GA²LEN)

Editor
Kiran Godse MD PhD FRCP (Glasg)
Professor of Dermatology
Dr DY Patil Medical College and Hospital
Navi Mumbai, Maharashtra, India

Associate Editor
Anant Patil
Dr DY Patil Medical College and Hospital
Navi Mumbai, Maharashtra, India

Foreword
Torsten Zuberbier

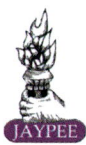

JAYPEE BROTHERS MEDICAL PUBLISHERS
The Health Sciences Publisher
New Delhi | London

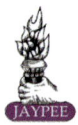 **Jaypee Brothers Medical Publishers (P) Ltd**

Headquarters

Jaypee Brothers Medical Publishers (P) Ltd
4838/24, Ansari Road, Daryaganj
New Delhi 110 002, India
Phone: +91-11-43574357
Fax: +91-11-43574314
Email: jaypee@jaypeebrothers.com

Overseas Office

J.P. Medical Ltd
83 Victoria Street, London
SW1H 0HW (UK)
Phone: +44 20 3170 8910
Fax: +44 (0)20 3008 6180
Email: info@jpmedpub.com

Website: www.jaypeebrothers.com
Website: www.jaypeedigital.com

© 2021, Jaypee Brothers Medical Publishers

The views and opinions expressed in this book are solely those of the original contributor(s)/author(s) and do not necessarily represent those of editor(s) of the book.

All rights reserved. No part of this publication may be reproduced, stored or transmitted in any form or by any means, electronic, mechanical, photocopying, recording or otherwise, without the prior permission in writing of the publishers.

All brand names and product names used in this book are trade names, service marks, trademarks or registered trademarks of their respective owners. The publisher is not associated with any product or vendor mentioned in this book.

Medical knowledge and practice change constantly. This book is designed to provide accurate, authoritative information about the subject matter in question. However, readers are advised to check the most current information available on procedures included and check information from the manufacturer of each product to be administered, to verify the recommended dose, formula, method and duration of administration, adverse effects and contraindications. It is the responsibility of the practitioner to take all appropriate safety precautions. Neither the publisher nor the author(s)/editor(s) assume any liability for any injury and/or damage to persons or property arising from or related to use of material in this book.

This book is sold on the understanding that the publisher is not engaged in providing professional medical services. If such advice or services are required, the services of a competent medical professional should be sought.

Every effort has been made where necessary to contact holders of copyright to obtain permission to reproduce copyright material. If any have been inadvertently overlooked, the publisher will be pleased to make the necessary arrangements at the first opportunity. The **CD/DVD-ROM** (if any) provided in the sealed envelope with this book is complimentary and free of cost. **Not meant for sale.**

Inquiries for bulk sales may be solicited at: jaypee@jaypeebrothers.com

Atopic Dermatitis and Pruritus: Interesting Cases / *Kiran Godse*

First Edition: **2021**

ISBN: 978-93-5152-238-6

Printed at: Samrat Offset Pvt. Ltd.

Contributors

Amina Mohamednoor Al-Obaidli
Department of Dermatology
Hamad Medical Corporation
Doha, Qatar

Akio Tanaka
Department of Dermatology
Graduate School of Biomedical
and Health Sciences
Hiroshima University
Hiroshima, Japan

Ana Paula Cusato-Ensina
CPAlpha Clinical Research and
Allergy Center
Barueri, São Paulo, Brazil

Anant Patil
Dr DY Patil Medical College
and Hospital
Navi Mumbai, Maharashtra, India

Andrzej Bożek
Department of Internal
Medicine, Dermatology and
Allergology
Medical University of Silesia in
Katowice, Poland

Angilieri L
Dermatology Unit, Fondazione
IRCCS Ca' Granda Ospedale
Maggiore Policlinico
Via Pace, 9, 20122
Milan, Italy

Barbara Rogala
Department of Internal
Medicine, Allergology and
Clinical Immunology
Medical University of Silesia in
Katowice, Poland

Bartłomiej Wawrzycki
Medical University of Lublin
Lublin, Poland

Berti E
Dermatology Unit, Fondazione
IRCCS Ca' Granda Ospedale
Maggiore Policlinico
Via Pace, 9, 20122, Milan, Italy
Department of Physiopathology
and Transplantation
Università degli Studi di Milano
Milan, Italy

Boneschi V
Dermatology Unit
Fondazione IRCCS Ca' Granda
Ospedale Maggiore Policlinico
Via Pace, 9, 20122, Milan, Italy

Célia Costa
Immunoallergology Department
Hospital de Santa Maria, Centro
Hospitalar Universitário Lisboa
Norte (CHULN)
Lisbon, Portugal

Charussri Leeyaphan
Department of Dermatology
Faculty of Medicine Siriraj
Hospital, Mahidol University
Bangkok, Thailand

Chuda Rujitharanawong
Department of Dermatology
Faculty of Medicine Siriraj
Hospital, Mahidol University
Bangkok, Thailand

Dorota Krasowska
Medical University of Lublin
Lublin, Poland

E Serra-Baldrich
Cutaneous Immuno-Allergy Unit
Department of Dermatology
Hospital Sant Pau, Universitat
Autònoma Barcelona
Spain

Elene Kakabadze
Center of Allergy and
Immunology
Tbilisi, Georgia

Eman Alsayed
Al-Rashed Allergy Center
Ministry of Health
Kuwait

Emek Kocatürk
Department of Dermatology
Koç University School of
Medicine
Istanbul, Turkey

Esra Saraç
Department of Dermatology
Koç University School of
Medicine, Istanbul, Turkey

Ethar Said Mohamed Al Hajri
University of Huddersfield
Huddersfield, United Kingdom

Fernanda Sales da Cunha
CPAlpha Clinical Research and
Allergy Center
Barueri, São Paulo, Brazil

Feroz K
Dr Feroz's Skin Care Clinic
Kannur, Kerala, India

Ferrucci S
Dermatology Unit, Fondazione
IRCCS Ca' Granda Ospedale
Maggiore Policlinico
Via Pace, 9, 20122
Milan, Italy

Gabriel Peres
Botucatu Medical School
State University of São Paulo
(FMB-UNESP)
Botucatu, São Paulo, Brazil

Gauri Godse
MGM Medical College
and Hospital
Navi Mumbai, Maharashtra, India

Giorgi Shengelidze
Center of Allergy and
Immunology
Tbilisi, Georgia

Germiniasi F
Dermatology Unit Fondazione
IRCCS Ca' Granda Ospedale
Maggiore Policlinico Via Pace
Milan, Italy
Department of Physiopathology
and Transplantation, Università
degli Studi di Milano, Milan, Italy

Guillet Carole
Allergy Unit
Department of Dermatology
University Hospital of Zürich
Zürich, Switzerland

Hajime Shindo
Shindo Dermatology and
Allergy Clinic
Hiroshima, Japan

Humaid A Al Wahshi
Immunologist and
Rheumatologist
Royal Hospital
Muscat, Oman

Iman Nasr
Immunologist and Allergist
Royal Hospital
Muscat, Oman

Jennifer Astrup Sørensen
Department of Dermatology
Bispebjerg Hospital
Copenhagen, Denmark

Jesper Grønlund Holm
Department of Dermatology
Bispebjerg Hospital
Copenhagen, Denmark

J Spertino
Cutaneous Immuno-Allergy Unit
Department of Dermatology
Hospital Sant Pau, Universitat
Autònoma Barcelona
Spain

Joanna Bartosińska
Medical University of Lublin
Poland

Jonathan A Bernstein
Bernstein Allergy Group Inc
Cincinnati, Ohio, United States
Division of Immunology/
Allergy Section, Department
of Internal Medicine, The
University of Cincinnati College
of Medicine
Cincinnati, Ohio, United States

Justin Greiwe
Bernstein Allergy Group Inc
Cincinnati, Ohio, United States
Division of Immunology/
Allergy Section, Department
of Internal Medicine, The
University of Cincinnati College
of Medicine
Cincinnati, Ohio, United States

Kanokvalai Kulthanan
Department of Dermatology
Faculty of Medicine Siriraj
Hospital, Mahidol University
Bangkok, Thailand

Kanyalak Munprom
Department of Dermatology
Faculty of Medicine Siriraj
Hospital, Mahidol University
Bangkok, Thailand

Ketevan Kvaratskhelia
Center of Allergy and
Immunology
Tbilisi, Georgia

Kiran Godse
Dr DY Patil Medical College
and Hospital
Navi Mumbai, Maharashtra, India

Sumanas Bunyaratavej
Department of Dermatology
Faculty of Medicine Siriraj
Hospital, Mahidol University
Bangkok, Thailand

Kolm Isabel
Allergy Unit
Department of Dermatology
University Hospital of Zürich
Zürich, Switzerland

Kripa Ajmera
Dr DY Patil Medical College
and Hospital
Navi Mumbai, Maharashtra, India

L Angileri
Department of Pathophysiology
and Transplantation
Dermatology Unit, IRCCS
Foundation Ca' Granda
Ospedale Maggiore Policlinico,
Milan, Italy

L Puig
Cutaneous Immuno-Allergy Unit
Department of Dermatology
Hospital Sant Pau, Universitat
Autònoma Barcelona, Spain

Lesia Rozłucka
Department of Internal
Medicine, Allergology and
Clinical Immunology
Medical University of Silesia in
Katowice, Poland

Line Brok Nørreslet
Bispebjerg University Hospital
Copenhagen, Denmark

Luis Felipe Ensina
CPAlpha Clinical Research and
Allergy Center
Barueri, São Paulo, Brazil

Maryam Ali Al-Nesf
Allergy and Clinical Immunology
Section, Department of Medicine
Hamad Medical Corporation
Doha, Qatar

Maia Gotua
Center of Allergy and
Immunology
Tbilisi, Georgia

Marisa Paulino
Immunoallergology Department
Hospital de Santa Maria, Centro
Hospitalar Universitário Lisboa
Norte (CHULN), Lisbon, Portugal

Michael Rudenko
The London Allergy and
Immunology Centre
London, United Kingdom

Michał Adamczyk
Medical University of Lublin
Poland

Michihiro Hide
Department of Dermatology
Graduate School of Biomedical
and Health Sciences
Hiroshima University
Hiroshima, Japan

Mona Al-Ahmad
Microbiology Department
Faculty of Medicine
Kuwait University, Kuwait
Al-Rashed Allergy Center
Ministry of Health
Kuwait

Nana Dolidze
Center of Allergy and
Immunology
Tbilisi, Georgia

Nino Lomidze
Center of Allergy and
Immunology
Tbilisi, Georgia

Nuttagarn Jantanapornchai
Department of Dermatology
Faculty of Medicine
Siriraj Hospital, Mahidol
University
Bangkok, Thailand

Omar Lupi
Serviço de Imunologia
do Hospital Universitário
Clementino Fraga Filho
(HUCFF-UFRJ)
Rio de Janeiro, Brazil

Paulo Ricardo Criado
ABC School of Medicine
Fundação Universitária do ABC
(FUABC), Santo André
São Paulo, Brazil

Penvadee Pattanaprichakul
Department of Dermatology
Faculty of Medicine Siriraj
Hospital, Mahidol University
Bangkok, Thailand

Prabha MP Liyanage
Medical officer
Internal Medicine Department
Royal Hospital
Muscat, Oman

Roberta Fachini Jardim Criado
ABC School of Medicine
Fundação Universitária do ABC
(FUABC)
Santo André, São Paulo, Brazil

Rosset Nina
Allergy Unit
Department of Dermatology
University Hospital of Zürich
Zürich, Switzerland

Rungsima Kiratiwongwan
Department of Dermatology
Faculty of Medicine Siriraj
Hospital, Mahidol University
Bangkok, Thailand

Ryo Saito
Department of Dermatology
Graduate School of Biomedical
and Health Sciences
Hiroshima University
Hiroshima, Japan

Salma Ahmed Taha
Allergy and Clinical Immunology
Section
Department of Medicine
Hamad Medical Corporation
Doha, Qatar

Schmid-Grendelmeier Peter
Allergy Unit
Department of Dermatology
University Hospital of Zürich
Zürich, Switzerland
Christine-Kühne Center for
Allergy research and Education
CK-CARE, Switzerland

Shamsa H Al Maawali
Internal Medicine Oman Medical
Speciality Board
Oman

Shunsuke Takahagi
Department of Dermatology
Graduate School of Biomedical
and Health Sciences
Hiroshima University
Hiroshima, Japan

Simon Francis Thomsen
Department of Biomedical
Sciences, University of
Copenhagen
Copenhagen, Denmark
Bispebjerg University Hospital
Copenhagen, Denmark

Solange Oliveira Rodrigues Valle
Serviço de Imunologia
do Hospital Universitário
Clementino Fraga Filho
(HUCFF-UFRJ)
Rio de Janeiro, Brazil

Steinmann Simona
Allergy Unit
Department of Dermatology
University Hospital of Zürich
Zürich, Switzerland

Sushrut Save
Dr Save's Clinic
Mumbai, Maharashtra, India

Tamara Theresia Lund
Bispebjerg University Hospital
Copenhagen, Denmark

Tavecchio S
Dermatology Unit Fondazione
IRCCS Ca' Granda Ospedale
Maggiore Policlinico
Via Pace, 9, 20122, Milan, Italy
Department of Physiopathology
and Transplantation, Università
degli Studi di Milano, Milan, Italy

Tejaswini Shekhar Sharma
Dr DY Patil Medical College
and Hospital
Navi Mumbai, Maharashtra, India

Tove Agner
Bispebjerg University Hospital
Copenhagen, Denmark

V Flores–Climent
Cutaneous Immuno-Allergy Unit
Department of Dermatology
Hospital Sant Pau, Universitat
Autònoma Barcelona, Spain

Vidal Haddad Jr
Dermatology and Radiotherapy
Department, Botucatu Medical
School, State University of São
Paulo (FMB-UNESP)
Botucatu, São Paulo, Brazil

Wafaa Talaat
Al-Rashed Allergy Center
Ministry of Health
Kuwait

Walter Belda Junior
Dermatology Department
Faculdade de Medicina da
Universidade de São Paulo
São Paulo, Brazil

Yasemin Topal Yüksel
Bispebjerg University Hospital
Copenhagen, Denmark

Foreword

In my role as the President of Global Allergy and Asthma European Network (GA^{2}LEN) and as Part of the Steering Committee of ADCARE, the Atopic Dermatitis Centres of Reference and Excellence, it is my great pleasure to write this foreword. Atopic dermatitis is a vexing disease with many different subtypes and a high variety of potential triggering factors which will always remain a challenge, not only for the practitioner but also for the patient as it can be a long journey to learn to live with the disease. Luckily, in the recent past, new developments and drug discoveries have occurred supporting especially those with severe atopic dermatitis, making their lives easier.

In this compilation of 30 cases (atopic dermatitis and pruritus), this book offers an insight into the sometimes-difficult diagnostic procedures as well as the variety of treatments which can help and support our patients. This book provides an interesting read for both general practitioners and specialists alike.

Eczema in general and atopic dermatitis as a disease is frequent in our modern world, especially so in urban areas with a high level of pollution. Allergies, as the most frequent comorbidity in atopic dermatitis, are still on the rise.

Last but not least, this book is also a prime example of how networking with centers of excellence aids the collection of interesting cases, thus supporting each other for a better understanding of the disease.

Torsten Zuberbier
President of GA^{2}LEN and as Part of the
Steering Committee of ADCARE
GA^{2}LEN ADCARE Network
www.ga2len-adcare.net

Preface

I am happy to present this book on *"Atopic Dermatitis and Pruritus: Interesting Cases"* to you.

This book is the result of extensive efforts from dermatologists all over the world. It contains 20 interesting cases related to Atopic Dermatitis and 10 interesting cases related to Pruritus from patients across the world. Expert authors from different countries have contributed to these cases.

I am sure readers will enjoy different perspectives on management of atopic dermatitis and pruritus around the world.

I must thank Dr Anant Patil for his significant contribution in editing and consistent follow-up and coordination with all international authors in collection of cases. I also thank Jaypee Brothers Medical Publishers (P) Ltd for supporting this initiative.

I wish to thank my family Dr Meenal, Dr Gauri and Atharva for supporting my academic activities.

Kiran Godse MD PhD FRCP (Glasg)
Professor of Dermatology
Dr DY Patil Medical College and Hospital
Navi Mumbai, Maharashtra, India

Contents

SECTION 1— INTERESTING CASES: ATOPIC DERMATITIS

Case 1: Severe Atopic Dermatitis in a Patient with a History of Renal Transplantation   3
Barbara Rogala, Lesia Rozłucka, Andrzej Bożek

Case 2: Recalcitrant Red Plaque in a Patient with Atopic Dermatitis   8
Chuda Rujitharanawong, Kanyalak Munprom, Rungsima Kiratiwongwan, Sumanas Bunyaratavej, Kanokvalai Kulthanan

Case 3: Successful Treatment of Prurigo Nodularis with Dupilumab in an Elderly Patient with Atopic Disease   11
Paulo Ricardo Criado, Roberta Fachini Jardim Criado

Case 4: Two Cases of Severe Adult-onset Atopic Dermatitis Responsive to Dupilumab   19
Justin Greiwe, Jonathan A Bernstein

Case 5: A Quality-of-life Game Changer: Treatment with Dupilumab in an Adult with Atopic Dermatitis   25
Line Brok Nørreslet, Yasemin Topal Yüksel, Tamara Theresia Lund, Tove Agner, Simon Francis Thomsen

Case 6: Refractory Atopic Dermatitis in a Young Male Patient: Course and Symptoms Following Start of Dupilumab   29
Tamara Theresia Lund, Line Brok Nørreslet, Yasemin Topal Yüksel, Tove Agner, Simon Francis Thomsen

Case 7: Erythrodermic Early Onset Atopic Dermatitis Clinically Mimicking Mycoses Fungoides/Sezary Disease   32
Ferrucci S, Tavecchio S, Angilieri L, Germiniasi F, Berti E, Boneschi V

Case 8: Food Allergy, Vaccination and Atopic Dermatitis Treatment in Children   35
Luis Felipe Ensina, Fernanda Sales da Cunha, Ana Paula Cusato-Ensina

Case 9: Do Not Miss Contact Allergy in Atopic Dermatitis Patients   38
Esra Saraç, Emek Kocatürk

Case 10:	Successful Treatment of Epidermolysis Bullosa Pruriginosa with Anti-IgE Therapy (Omalizumab): A Case Report and 4 Years Follow-up *Salma Ahmed Taha, Maryam Ali Al-Nesf, Amina Mohamednoor Al-Obaidli*	44
Case 11:	The Cause Behind Multiple Drug Hypersensitivity Reactions in a Patient with Atopic Dermatitis *Iman Nasr, Shamsa H Al Maawali, Prabha MP Liyanage*	48
Case 12:	Severe Atopic Dermatitis: Fast Effectiveness and Safety of Dupilumab *Marisa Paulino, Célia Costa*	52
Case 13:	Role of Patch Testing in Atopic Dermatitis *Michael Rudenko*	55
Case 14:	Eczema Herpeticum in a Patient with Atopic Dermatitis during Treatment with Selective JAK1 Inhibitor: A Case Report *Michał Adamczyk, Bartłomiej Wawrzycki, Joanna Bartosińska, Dorota Krasowska*	57
Case 15:	Dupilumab-induced Face Dermatitis in Patients with Adult-onset Atopic Dermatitis and Severe Asthma *Mona Al-Ahmad, Eman Alsayed, Wafaa Talaat*	62
Case 16:	Dupilumab in the Treatment of Severe Atopic Dermatitis and Eczema Herpeticum Refractory to Systemic Treatment *Omar Lupi, Solange Oliveira Rodrigues Valle*	65
Case 17:	Red Face during Dupilumab Therapy *E Serra-Baldrich, V Flores–Climent, J Spertino, L Puig*	69
Case 18:	A Case Report of a Patient with Refractory Severe Atopic Dermatitis and Extremely High Total Serum IgE Levels Treated with High Doses of Omalizumab in Combination with Conventional Therapy *Maia Gotua, Nino Lomidze, Giorgi Shengelidze, Elene Kakabadze, Ketevan Kvaratskhelia, Nana Dolidze*	72
Case 19:	Atopic Dermatitis in Skin of Color *Kiran Godse, Kripa Ajmera, Gauri Godse, Anant Patil*	76
Case 20:	Herbal Preparations Causing Irritation in a Patient with Atopic Dermatitis: A Case Report *Tejaswini Shekhar Sharma, Gauri Godse, Anant Patil, Feroz K*	79

SECTION 2— INTERESTING CASES: PRURITUS

Case 1: Long-term Efficacy and Safety of Dupilumab in Prurigo Nodularis: A Case Report — 85
Germiniasi F, Tavecchio S, L Angileri, Berti E, Ferrucci S

Case 2: Generalized Purpuric Macules with Intense Pruritus: A Single Case Report — 89
Chuda Rujitharanawong, Nuttagarn Jantanapornchai, Charussri Leeyaphan, Penvadee Pattanaprichakul, Kanokvalai Kulthanan

Case 3: Importance of Dietary History in the Presence of a Biopsy Suggestive of Urticarial Vasculitis — 93
Iman Nasr, Humaid A Al Wahshi, Shamsa H Al Maawali, Ethar Said Mohamed Al Hajri

Case 4: Chronic Suffering from Undiagnosed Generalized Itching, Papules, and Plaques: The Relief Impact of a Single Dermoscope Examination — 98
Gabriel Peres, Vidal Haddad Jr, Roberta Fachini Jardim Criado, Walter Belda Junior, Paulo Ricardo Criado

Case 5: A Case of Pruritus with Symptomatic Dermographism Previously Treated as Eczema — 104
Ryo Saito, Hajime Shindo, Shunsuke Takahagi, Akio Tanaka, Michihiro Hide

Case 6: Immediate and Long-lasting Resolution of Pruritus and Skin Lesions by Targeting the IL-5 Receptor — 107
Guillet Carole, Steinmann Simona, Rosset Nina, Kolm Isabel, Schmid-Grendelmeier Peter

Case 7: An Unexpected Cause of Symptomatic Dermographism: Scabies — 112
Esra Saraç, Emek Kocatürk

Case 8: Intensive Pruritus, Excoriations and Inflammatory Papules Masking Dermatitis Herpetiformis — 117
Maia Gotua, Elene Kakabadze

Case 9: Diagnosis and In Vivo Detection of *Sarcoptes Scabiei* by Dermoscopy — 121
Sushrut Save, Kiran Godse

Case 10: Prurigo Nodularis Treated Successfully with Dupilumab: Case Report and Review of the Literature — 124
Jennifer Astrup Sørensen, Jesper Grønlund Holm, Simon Francis Thomsen

Index — 131

SECTION

1

Interesting Cases: Atopic Dermatitis

CASE 1

Severe Atopic Dermatitis in a Patient with a History of Renal Transplantation

Barbara Rogala, Lesia Rozłucka, Andrzej Bożek

CASE PRESENTATION

A 22-year-old Caucasian man was urgently admitted to the Dermatology and Allergology Department due to generalized erythroderma in the course of severe atopic dermatitis (AD). The patient reported increasing skin deterioration for several weeks before hospitalization, accompanied by a mild increase of temperature. Exacerbation of the symptoms, by his own admission, coincided with a prolonged (several weeks) high exposure to dust and mold (old and damp apartment). The patient did not associate deterioration of his health status with either food or medication intake. He emphasized that the symptoms intensified despite the medication recommended during the last visit in the Outpatient Dermatology Clinic.

COURSE OF ILLNESS

The patient has suffered from atopic dermatitis (AD) since the age of 3 years. The course of the disease varied with periods of remission and exacerbation. Initial mild form of the disease progressed periodically to moderate form, treated in the Outpatient Dermatology and Allergology Clinic at the place of residence. During the early childhood, the patient noted a significant relationship between the exacerbation of skin lesions and the consumption of chicken eggs and milk. Later, he did not observe any adverse food-related reactions.

Since 12 years old, the patient suffered from periodic allergic rhinitis during the tree dusting season and was treated symptomatically with antihistamine drugs. During this period, the patient presented signs and symptoms of bronchial asthma. Exacerbations during the fall-winter period were periodically treated with inhaled corticosteroids and β2-mimetics. Presently, the patient does not experience symptoms of asthma.

Additionally, the patient was diagnosed with nephroangiosclerosis and renal hypertension in the early childhood. In 2006, the right kidney transplant was performed due to the progressive vascular sclerosis with increasing kidney failure and arterial hypertension. The postoperative course was uneventful. The patient received chronic, immunosuppressive therapy (tacrolimus and mycophenolate mofetil), which was constantly supervised by the nephrologist.

Since 2013, there was a significant worsening of the AD symptoms, despite continued use of topical corticosteroids, emollients, and oral antihistamines. An addition of prednisone in a dose of 10–15 mg daily allowed for a relative control of the disease symptoms. Immunosuppressants were administered chronically: Tacrolimus 3 mg daily and mycophenolate mofetil 750 mg daily.

First Hospitalization

In November 2019, the patient was hospitalized in the Department of Dermatology and Allergology due to exacerbation of AD. Assessment of skin condition showed 65–70 points according to the SCORAD (SCORing Atopic Dermatitis) scale. A laboratory test revealed an increased C-reactive protein level, leukocytosis ($12.51 \times 10^3/\mu L$), eosinophilia (7.8%), and increased total immunoglobulin E (IgE) level (2,500 IU/mL); serum levels of IgA, IgM, IgG, and c1q complex were within the normal. The results of aeroallergen and food-specific IgE concentration are presented in **Table 1**.

Autoimmune profiles (ANA1, ANA2, ANA3) were negative. Genetic testing revealed mutation of the filaggrin gene *2282del4* as a heterozygote. In cultures from skin lesions, nose and throat, a significant increase of *Staphylococcus aureus* was found. An antibiotic was applied according to the antibiogram (amoxicillin 3 × 1 g/day) as well as prednisone 15 mg/day and loratadine 2 × 20 mg/day. In addition, external treatment was modified to include first-line topical corticosteroids (clobetasol propionate) followed by tacrolimus (0.1%) ointment, which resulted in a clinical improvement. The immunosuppressive therapy was continued without change of drug dosage, all in consultation with the nephrological transplant center.

TABLE 1: Serum-specific IgE concentration of inhalant and food allergens (Polycheck) and their interpretation.

Lp.	Allergen	sIgE (kU/L)	Class
Inhalant panel			
1.	Sweet vernal grass pollen	83.00	5
2.	Cocksfoot pollen	68.00	5
3.	Timothy Grass pollen	94.00	5
4.	Rye pollen	80.00	5
5.	Alder pollen	66.00	5
6.	Birch pollen	67.00	5
7.	Hazel pollen	27.00	4
8.	White oak pollen	8.20	3
9.	Ragweed pollen	0.54	1
10.	Mugwort pollen	0.59	1
11.	Plantain pollen	91.00	5
12.	*Dermatophagoides pteronyssinus*	74.00	5
13.	*Dermatophagoides farinae*	≥100	6
14.	Cat epithelia	91.00	5
15.	Dog epithelia	≥100	6
16.	Horse epithelia	<0.15	0
17.	*Penicillium notatum*	4.30	3
18.	*Cladosporium herbarum*	0.90	2
19.	*Aspergillus fumigatus*	2.40	2
20.	*Alternaria alternata*	2.90	2
21.	CCD marker	2.70	2
Food panel			
1.	Egg white	21.00	4
2.	Egg yolk	5.10	3
3.	Milk	<0.15	0
4.	Baker's yeast	1.10	2
5.	Wheat flour	3.80	3

Continued

Continued

Lp.	Allergen	sIgE (kU/L)	Class
6.	Rye flour	2.70	2
7.	Rice	2.80	2
8.	Soybean	<0.15	0
9.	Peanut	0.40	1
10.	Hazelnut	12.20	3
11.	Almond	0.28	0
12.	Apple	1.10	2
13.	Kiwi	0.22	0
14.	Apricot	0.36	0
15.	Tomato	0.61	1
16.	Carrot	0.80	2
17.	Potato	1.30	2
18.	Celery	3.20	2
19.	Codfish	<0.15	0
20.	Crab	7.90	3
21.	CCD marker	3.20	2

sIgE (kU/L)	Class	Interpretation
<0.35	0	No specific antibody detectable
0.35–<0.7	1	Very weak antibody concentration
0.7–<3.5	2	Weak antibody concentration
3.5–<17.5	3	Clear antibody concentration
17.5–<50	4	Strong antibody concentration
50–<100	5	Very strong antibody concentration
>100	6	Extremely high antibody concentration

(CCD: cross-reactive carbohydrate determinant; sIgE: specific immunoglobulin E)

Due to a significant improvement of the patient's skin condition, the patient was discharged from the hospital on a reduced dose of prednisone to 10 mg/day. In the following 2 months, the disease stabilized; there was no itching of the skin and a reduction of skin lesions' size was noted.

Second Hospitalization

Sudden exacerbation of the disease took place in January 2020. The patient was readmitted to the Department of Dermatology and Allergology. The physical findings on admission were as follows: Generalized extensive erythema (SCORAD 90), exudative lesions with numerous erosions, very strong burning and hyperalgesia of the skin, and temperature rise. No other significant deviation in the physical examination was identified. The immunosuppressive treatment was continued according to the scheme recommended by the nephrologist—mycophenolate mofetil 2 × 500 mg/day and 2 mg of tacrolimus in the morning and 1 mg in the evening as well as antibiotic therapy (initially amoxicillin + clavulanic acid 3 times 1 g/day orally and then cefuroxime, initially 2 times 750 mg and then 2 times 1.5 g intravenously), antihistamine (bilastine 20 mg twice a day) and 4 mg of dexamethasone intravenous twice a day.

The external treatment was intensified (cholesterol ointment, boric acid compresses, emollients and mometasone furoate). After the nephrology consultation, a decision to replace mycophenolate mofetil with methotrexate 15 mg/day was made.

After the third dose of methotrexate a dry, paroxysmal cough, increased body temperature (37.8°C), laryngitis, stomach ache, and diarrhea (four to six stools per day) were recorded. Suspecting a *Clostridium difficile* infection, the specific test was performed. A presence of the antigen *Clostridium difficile*, in the absence of the toxin, was identified.

Nevertheless, due to the clinical presentation, vancomycin (250 mg/day for 10 days) was administered. Dexamethasone was set aside; prednisone 20 mg/day was used together with bilastine 20 mg twice a day. Skin care practices were maintained (cholesterol

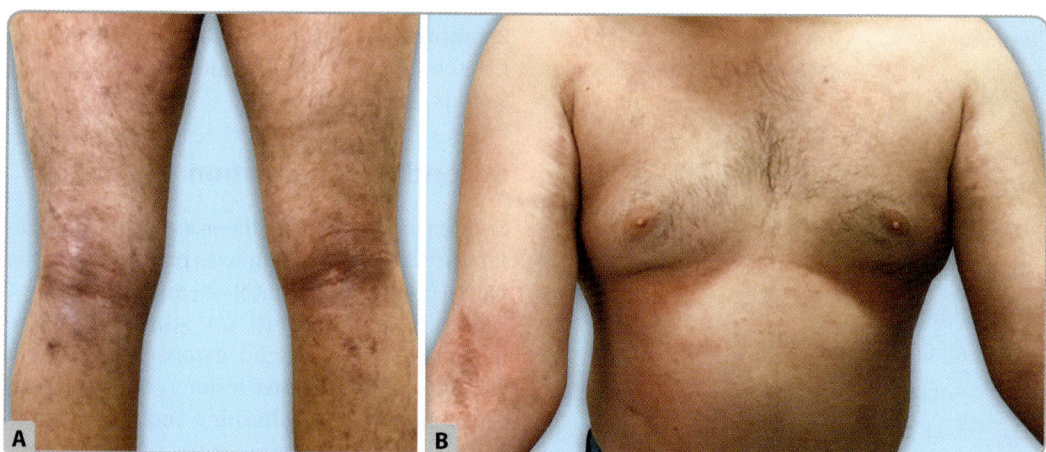

FIGS. 1A AND B: Patient's skin condition during the latest visit in the hospital outpatient clinic.

ointment, emollients cooling ointment with hydrocortisone) and hypertension treatment was continued (amlodipine 10 mg/day, ramipril 2.5 mg/day). Due to the cough, nebulization of budesonide 2 times 1.0/day was given. The immunosuppressive treatment was continued. Diarrhea and cough subsided within 48 hours.

A significant improvement of the skin condition was noted: From a generalized form to regional lesions on the lower limbs, elbow flexion areas as well as neck and face (SCORAD: 60–65 points).

Follow-up

The patient received the treatment as above, with gradual reduction of prednisone to 10 mg/day (other drugs, including the remaining immunosuppressive regimen, as during the hospitalization). Topical treatment included mometasone furoate, tacrolimus and fludrocortisone acetate (on face) and emollients. Presently, the patient is constantly monitored in the Hospital Outpatient Clinic. Figure 1 presents the patient's skin condition during the last control visit.

DISCUSSION

Atopic dermatitis is a chronic inflammatory skin disorder. The pathophysiology of the disease is not completely understood. It is a complex interplay between immune dysregulation, environmental and infectious agents, and disturbed skin function.[1] Although our patient demonstrates a high degree of sensitization to aeroallergens, it does not explain completely the aggravation of the disease, which turns into severe after several years of renal transplantation. Having experienced exacerbation of his skin disorder in response to house mites and molds, the patient has taken avoidance measures. It can be assumed that the immunosuppressive drugs administered after the renal transplantation might be responsible for the worsening of the disease.[2,3]

Nevertheless, it is worth noticing that post-transplant immunosuppressive agents are frequently advised in the management of patients with severe AD.[4-7]

In spite of the application of the commonly recommended treatment, which included topical emollients/moisturizers, corticosteroids, and calcineurin inhibitors, the condition of the patient's AD exacerbated and became complicated with erythroderma. The condition of the skin significantly improved following the application of antibiotics and prednisone. This strongly implicates skin infection as the main cause of the AD exacerbation. Filaggrin mutation, which was confirmed in the patient, is a known factor predisposing to skin superinfection.[8] However, the effect of chronic immunosuppressive therapy on the exacerbation of AD cannot be completely excluded.

CONCLUSION

Patients suffering from severe AD and concomitant severe medical disorders should remain under constant control of several specialists.

KEY MESSAGES

- Although IgE-mediated sensitization to the airborne allergens is an important feature of the AD pathophysiology, it is not the sole factor of its underlying mechanism.
- IgE-mediated sensitization may have limited clinical relevance, particularly in the severe stage of the disease.
- Severe exacerbation of the AD may be observed in some groups of patients in spite of the application of the recommended treatment (topical corticosteroids and optimal care practices) and allergens' avoidance.
- The skin infection, as a causative factor of severe AD exacerbation, should be taken into account, particularly in patients with filaggrin mutation and concomitant, not only atopic, diseases.

REFERENCES

1. Wollenberg A, Barbarot S, Bieber T, Christen-Zaech S, Deleuran M, Fin-Wagner A, et al. Consensus-based European guidelines for treatment of atopic eczema (atopic dermatitis) in adults and children: part II. J Eur Acad Dermatology Venereol. 2018;32:850-78.
2. Arikan C, Kilic M, Tokat Y, Aydogdu S. Allergic disease after pediatric liver transplantation with systemic tacrolimus and cyclosporine a therapy. Transplant Proc. 2003;35:3039-41.
3. Granot E, Yakobovich E, Bardenstein R. Tacrolimus immunosuppression - An association with asymptomatic eosinophilia and elevated total and specific IgE levels. Pediatr Transplant. 2006;10:690-3.
4. Murray ML, Cohen JB. Mycophenolate mofetil therapy for moderate to severe atopic dermatitis. Clin Exp Dermatol. 2007;32:23-7.
5. Phan K, Smith SD. Mycophenolate mofetil and atopic dermatitis: systematic review and meta-analysis. J Dermatolog Treat. 2019;1-5.
6. Keaney TC, Bhutani T, Sivanesan P, Bandow GD, Weinstein SB, Chenung LCC, et al. Open-label, pilot study examining sequential therapy with oral tacrolimus and topical tacrolimus for severe atopic dermatitis. J Am Acad Dermatol. 2012;67:636-41.
7. Lyakhovitsky A, Barzilai A, Heyman R, Baum S, Amichai B, Solomon M, et al. Low-dose methotrexate treatment for moderate-to-severe atopic dermatitis in adults. J Eur Acad Dermatology Venereol. 2010;24:43-9.
8. Clausen ML, Edslev SM, Andersen PS, Clemmensen K, Krogfelt KA, Agner T. *Staphylococcus aureus* colonization in atopic eczema and its association with filaggrin gene mutations. Br J Dermatol. 2017;177:1394-400.

CASE 2

Recalcitrant Red Plaque in a Patient with Atopic Dermatitis

Chuda Rujitharanawong, Kanyalak Munprom, Rungsima Kiratiwongwan, Sumanas Bunyaratavej, Kanokvalai Kulthanan

CASE PRESENTATION

A 6-year-old Thai boy with atopic dermatitis (AD) presented with a history of progressive itchy rash at the right side of his face for 1 month. He was diagnosed as AD flare-up at another hospital, and he was treated with oral prednisolone 10 mg/day for 1 week together with topical mometasone furoate-cream. The lesion initially improved, but then it began to gradually spread across his right cheek all the way to his nose. He had no history of pet contact.

Physical examination revealed a well-circumscribed, erythematous, scaly plaque on the right cheek, right eyelid, and nose (**Fig. 1**).

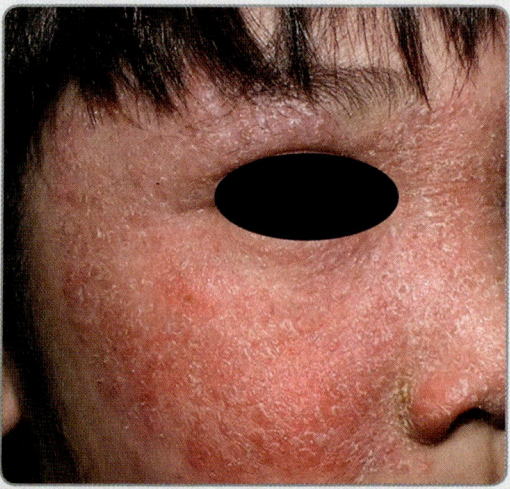

FIG. 1: A 6-year-old Thai boy with atopic dermatitis presented with a history of progressive itchy rash at the right side of his face for 1 month.

No rash was observed on any other part of his body and there were no other symptoms. Skin scraping for potassium hydroxide microscopic examination revealed positive branching septate hyphae with arthrospores and fungal vellus hair involvement as ectothrix invasion (**Fig. 2**).

Fungal culture was positive for *Trichophyton mentagrophytes*. He was diagnosed as AD with tinea incognito, and he was treated with oral fluconazole 200 mg/week for 3 weeks together with topical sertaconazole cream once daily. The lesion subsided with residual postinflammatory hyperpigmentation at the affected area.

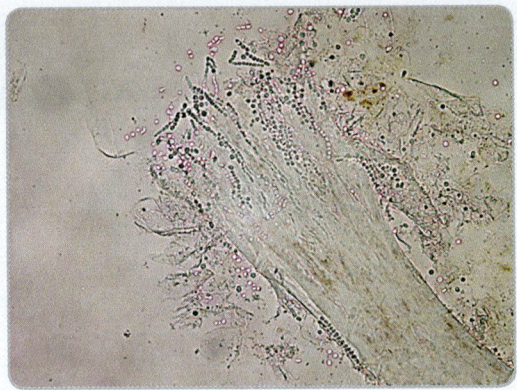

FIG. 2: Potassium hydroxide microscopic examination demonstrated positive branching septate hyphae with arthrospores and fungal vellus hair involvement as ectothrix invasion.

DISCUSSION

Atopic dermatitis (AD) is a chronic relapsing inflammatory skin disease. The common clinical presentations include dry skin, pruritus, and eczematous skin lesion with age-specific distribution. AD is accompanied by breakdown of the skin barrier due to dry skin and repetitive scratching, which leads to immune dysfunction that increases susceptibility to invasion by microorganisms that can cause cutaneous infection.[1,2] To reduce inflammation, topical corticosteroids are commonly prescribed to treat AD flare-up.[3] However, an adverse effect of topical corticosteroid use is local immunity suppression, which can increase the risk of infection.[3] In this patient, the skin lesion was a unilateral facial plaque. Our patient initially demonstrated a good clinical response to topical corticosteroid treatment, but flare-ups began to occur during ongoing treatment. We then reevaluated to determine if his skin lesion was a steroid-unresponsive disease, such as tinea incognito, or if he was allergic to one or more of the components of the topical corticosteroid. The morphology of the skin lesion was changed with ill-defined border and intense redness. Mycological investigation should be done. If the mycological result was negative, patch testing should be performed to exclude allergic contact dermatitis due to the components of topical corticosteroid. However, in our case, the result of potassium hydroxide microscopic examination was positive and tinea incognito was diagnosed.

Tinea incognito is a tinea infection that is modified by inappropriate topical corticosteroid application that interrupts local immunity and promotes fungal growth. Tinea incognito is sometimes difficult to diagnosis due to its often atypical appearance. The most common organisms that cause fungal skin infection on the face are zoophilic dermatophytes, including *Microsporum canis*, *T. rubrum*, or *T. mentagrophytes*.[4] Most patients infected with a zoophilic dermatophyte reported having a history of direct contact with animals. Although this patient denied any history of animal contact, indirect animal contact and microorganism contamination in clothes or household environment are other possible causes.[5]

Atopic dermatitis patients with fungal infection commonly have more severe lesions that are more difficult to diagnose, which is what was observed in our case. The use of topical corticosteroids and excoriation may be predisposing factors for microorganism invasion into the deeper part of the skin resulting in tinea of vellus hair.[6] Systemic antifungal treatment is recommended for tinea of vellus hair, and the outcome of treatment is usually favorable.[7] Similarly, our patient had a good clinical response to oral fluconazole synergist and topical sertaconazole.

CONCLUSION

Dry skin and impaired barrier function in patients with AD can lead to increased susceptibility to dermatophyte infection. Clinical presentation may sometimes resemble AD flare-up, which can lead to misdiagnosis and treatment with corticosteroids. In patients with atypical and/or refractory AD lesion, dermatologists should have a high index of suspicion for AD with tinea incognito, so mycological investigation should be performed to exclude this condition.

ACKNOWLEDGEMENT

The authors gratefully acknowledge the parents of the child described in this report for permitting us to disclose details relating to his case.

CONFLICT OF INTEREST DECLARATION

All authors declare no personal or professional conflicts of interest relating to any aspect of this case report.

FUNDING DISCLOSURE

This was an unfunded study.

KEY MESSAGE

- Tinea infection can present as an atopic dermatitis-like lesion in patients with atopic dermatitis.

REFERENCES

1. Faergemann J. Atopic dermatitis and fungi. Clin Microbiol Rev. 2002;15:545-63.
2. Ren Z, Silverberg JI. Association of atopic dermatitis with bacterial, fungal, viral, and sexually transmitted skin infections. Dermatitis. 2020;31:157-64.
3. Mounsey SJ, Agius E. Atopic dermatitis. Br J Hosp Med (Lond). 2017;78:C183-7.
4. Lange M, Jasiel-Walikowska E, Nowicki R, Bykowska B. Tinea incognito due to *Trichophyton mentagrophytes*. Mycoses. 2010;53:455-7.
5. Bunyaratavej S, Sombatmaithai S, Muanprasat C, Chularojanamontri L, Kulthanan K. Zoophilic dermatophytosis: A study of closed contact cases. Thai J Dermatol. 2008;24:194-207.
6. Kurian A, Haber RM. Tinea corporis gladiatorum presenting as a majocchi granuloma. ISRN Dermatol. 2011;2011:767589.
7. Gomez-Moyano E, Crespo-Erchiga V. Tinea of vellus hair: an indication for systemic antifungal therapy. Br J Dermatol. 2010;163:603-6.

CASE 3

Successful Treatment of Prurigo Nodularis with Dupilumab in an Elderly Patient with Atopic Disease

Paulo Ricardo Criado, Roberta Fachini Jardim Criado

CASE PRESENTATION

An 87-year-old man with Fitzpatrick's skin phototype IV with systemic arterial hypertension (SAH) and benign prostate hyperplasia (BPH) presented to our clinic with multiple hyperpigmented, lichenified papules and nodules, extremely pruritic, symmetrically distributed on face (**Figs. 1A** to **I**), upper and lower limbs, and trunk (**Figs. 1** and **2**). On her frontal area, subacute and chronic eczema was present during the physical examination. Palms and soles, besides the genital areas, were unaffected. No lymphadenopathy was observed on palpation in cervical, supraclavicular, and axillary areas or inguinal regions. Hepatomegaly and splenomegaly were absent. General blood tests were presented during the consultation which revealed a normal total blood cell count (except mild eosinophilia, 5% of total white blood cells), blood glucose levels, urea, creatinine, total cholesterol and triglycerides, total prostatic-specific antigen (PSA), and thyroid hormone levels, and stool tests were conducted as well. The total immunoglobulin E (IgE) serum level was 2,405 kU/L, and *Toxocara canis* serology was negative.

The clinical diagnosis of prurigo nodularis (PN) associated with adult AD was established.

The patient noticed suffer from these lesions and intensive itching during the last 4 years. 2 weeks ago, he developed a herpes-zoster eruption on the left abdomen. There is a history of allergic rhinitis in the past years. He treated his SAH with amlodipine and BPH using dutasteride plus tamsulosin for several years. He also noticed symptoms of anxiety and depression. Besides the uncontrolled itching, another remarkable complaint was the loss of sleep for several months. No history of familial pruritus was reported.

During the last 3 years, the patient had been treated by other physicians with several topical and systemic agents: Topical clobetasol, mometasone furoate, and intralesional triamcinolone (10 mg/mL); mirtazapine, pregabalin, hydroxyzine, and methotrexate (15 mg/week for 6 months); oral cyclosporine (4 mg/kg/day for several months); and prednisone (60 mg/day for 6 months), and posterior tapering off the doses until corticosteroid withdrawal. Several adverse effects with these medications were reported during the consultation including fatigue, uncontrolled

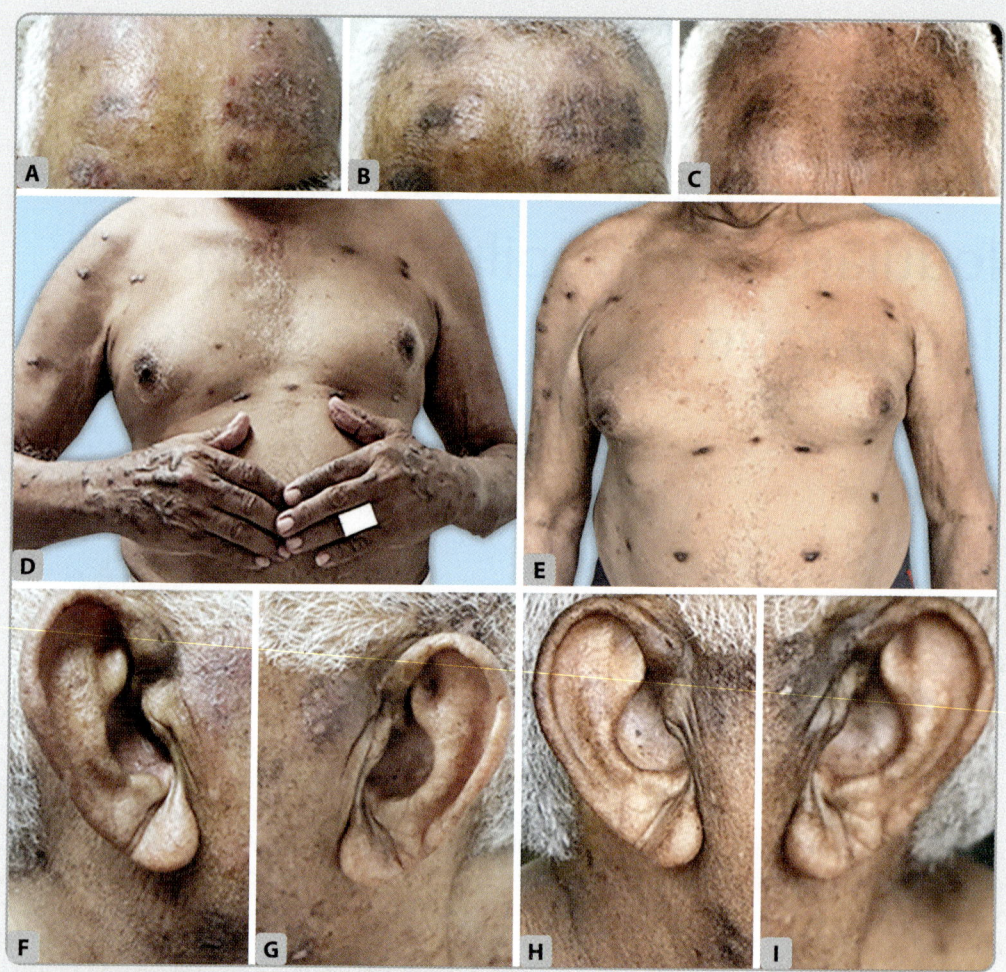

FIGS. 1A TO I: Evolution of the cutaneous lesions in our patient before and after Dupilumab treatment. (A) The frontal area during the first consultation showed erythematous-desquamative mild infiltrated plaques; (B) 1 month after the induction dose (600 mg) and the second dose of 300 mg; (C) the same frontal area after 4 months of the treatment onset showing only residual hyperchromic macules; (D) trunk at the first consultation demonstrating several infiltrated hyperpigmented nodules; (E) trunk after 4 months of treatment revealing less infiltrated lesions and residual hyperchromia; (F) and (G) erythema, papules, and nodules infiltrated around the ears; (H) and (I) after 4 months under treatment, the same area demonstrated only hyperchromic residual macules.

SAH, dizziness, and nausea and all these drugs were ineffective to control the pruritus and the development of new lesions in our patient.

Two cutaneous biopsies were collected previously of the frontal area and the right forearm, respectively. The first biopsy of a clinically acute/subacute eczematous lesion on face showed on optical microscopy in sectional skin fragments stained by hematoxylin-eosin (HE) a spongiotic epidermis with a lymphohistiocytic inflammatory dermal infiltrate in the perivascular dermal vessels with numerous eosinophils. In the second skin biopsy (forearm), there was chronic dermatitis with the compact hyperkeratotic epidermis, parakeratosis foci, and irregular acanthosis. Dermal fibrosis was present. Both skin samples were representative of the eczema spectrum.

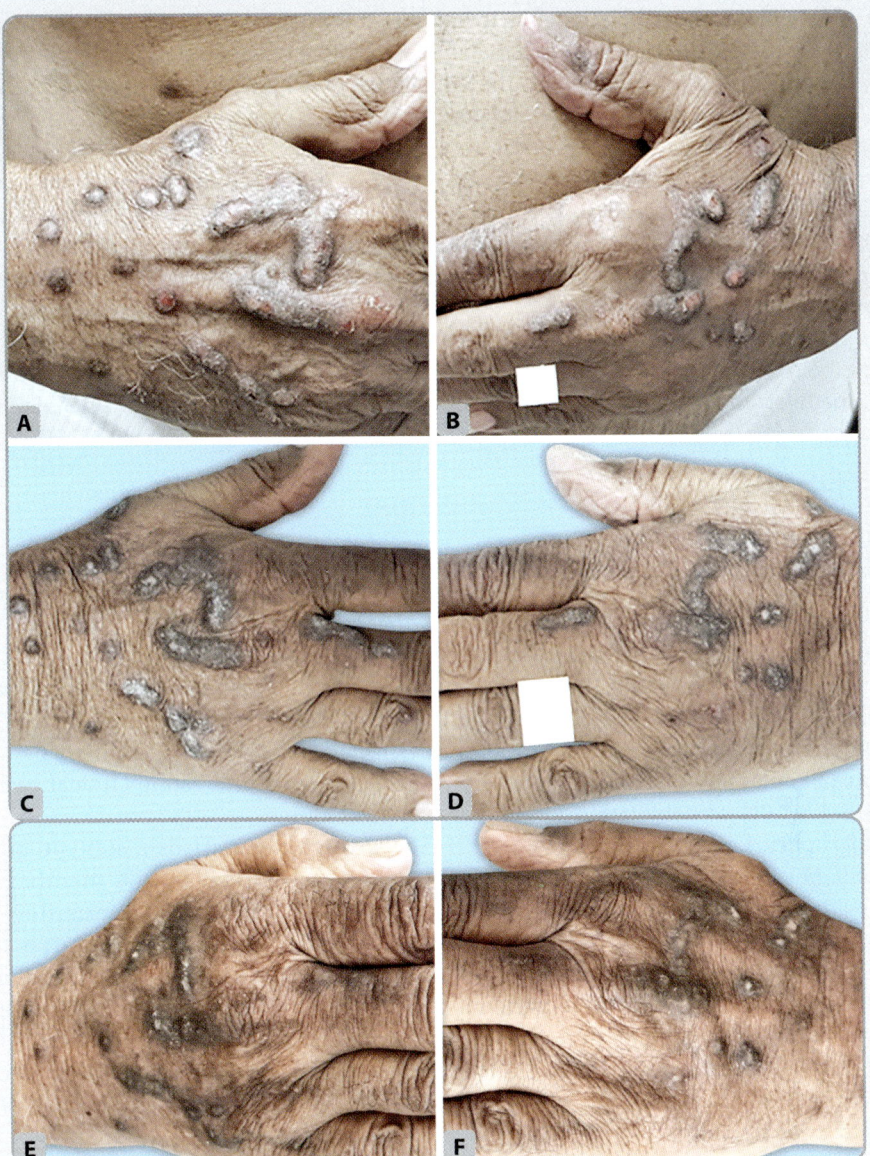

FIGS. 2A TO F: The sequential evolution of the hyperkeratotic infiltrated and excoriated isolated or confluent nodules on the patient's hands. (A) Right-hand and (B) left-hand aspects at the initial consultation (observe erosions and excoriations over nodules). (C) and (D) Less excoriated lesions at the end of the first treatment month with dupilumab; (E) and (F) after 4 months of dupilumab monotherapy, when the infiltrated and hyperkeratotic nodules showed an expressive regression and no erosion or excoriation was observed.

Take in count the previous failure treatments for his diseases, his age, and potentially the dangerous adverse effects of other immunosuppressive drugs such as azathioprine or mycophenolate mofetil, especially in this clinical scenario of several epidemic diseases in Brazil, such as dengue, zika virus, chikungunya infections, and others. We discussed with the patient and his family the off-label use of Dupilumab for PN, and the patient agreed with this treatment. During the first consultation, we applied the Visual Analogue Scale (VAS) for pruritus that resulted in a value of 10 (0 = no pruritus; <3 = mild pruritus; ≥3–<7 = moderate pruritus; ≥7–<9 = severe pruritus, and VAS ≥9 = very severe pruritus).

Dupilumab therapy was subsequently initiated, 600-mg subcutaneous injection at week 0 followed by 300-mg subcutaneous injection every 2 weeks. After 1 month of therapy (induction doses of 600 and 300 mg after 2 weeks), the VAS for pruritus was noticed as a value = 2 (0 = no pruritus; <3 = mild pruritus; ≥3–<7 = moderate pruritus; ≥7–<9 = severe pruritus, and VAS ≥9 = very severe pruritus).

The patient rapidly achieved decreased pruritus and expressive improvement of his cutaneous lesions albeit not full skin clearance over the last 4 months (decrease of the acute/subacute eczema, papules, and nodules subsequently shown in **Figs. 1** and **2**). He is off all other medications for pruritus. No adverse effects from Dupilumab monotherapy were reported.

DISCUSSION

Prurigo nodularis (PN), formerly named as prurigo nodular of Hyde, is a highly pruriginous chronic disease composed by the presence of several, usually symmetrically distributed, erythematous or brown-black hyperkeratotic and erosive papules and nodules, due to excoriations on skin.[1] PN is a debilitating dermatosis that usually appears at 40–50 years old.

In 1980, Miyachi et al.[2] studied 24 patients with PN with ages ranging from 12 to 79 years (mean age 31 years), and 16 (66.6%) had a positive personal and/or family history of atopic disorders, and often in these patients, the AD (45.6%) was more frequently found than asthma (12.5%) or allergic rhinitis (8.3%). These authors suggested that although emotional stress and repeated scratching have been implicated as contributory factors, the etiology of PN still remained to be determinate, but their impression was that PN occurred mainly in the patients with atopic background.[2] Miyachi et al.[2] speculated that one of the reasons why PN occurs more readily in atopic individuals is because they are more sensitive to insect bites or other scratching-provoking triggers causing itching on the skin, i.e., patients with atopic diathesis. These factors usually lead to compulsive scratching resulting in a verrucous appearance of the eruption.

Often, PN presents in the elderly and the traditional therapies used to treat this condition may conduct for potential dangerous adverse effects related to liver or kidney function in these patients. New therapies, with less potential adverse effects, must be tried for PN, especially for children and elderly patients. We are adding an interesting clinical case in this clinical setting.

Prurigo nodularis is a subtype of chronic prurigo as defined by the members of the European Academy of Dermatology and Venereology (EADV) Task Force Pruritus group, in which a neuronal sensitization to itch develops an itch-scratch cycle.[3] The debate on the nature of PN was initiated over >100 years ago after the first description of this condition by Hyde.[4] Several conditions have been described in association with PN, as listed in **Box 1**.[3-5]

Our patient, due to his personal history of rhinitis, peripheral blood eosinophilia, and elevated total IgE serum levels, is included among the distinct inflammatory disorders in association with PN, particularly AD, where PN may coexist with inflammatory dermatosis (in this patient, chronic eczema on neck and face) or continue after their cessation.[6] This association is sometimes described in terms such as "*pruriginous atopic eczema*," reflecting the synchronism and biological interconnection between both conditions.[1]

> **BOX 1: Distinct conditions related to prurigo nodularis.**
> - Atopic dermatitis (most frequent)
> - Cutaneous T-cell lymphoma
> - Lichen planus
> - Incipient bullous pemphigoid (direct immunofluorescence for diagnosis is indicated)[3]
> - Chronic kidney failure (10% of hemodialysis patients)[4]
> - Diabetes mellitus
> - HIV infection
> - Neuropathic diseases (damage to cutaneous or extracutaneous nerves, as related to postherpetic neuralgia or neuropathic pruritus, e.g., brachioradial pruritus, mainly localized in the dermatome C5/C6)
> - Psychiatric disorders (depression, anxiety, tactile hallucinations, skin-picking disorder of the skin without primarily perceiving pruritus)
> - Localized prurigo nodularis due to leg venous insufficiency[3]
> - Intense xerosis[5]
> - Liver diseases (chronic hepatitis B, hepatitis C, primary biliary cholangitis, chronic autoimmune cholestatic hepatitis)[5]
> - Thyroid disease[5]
> - Internal malignancies (especially non-Hodgkin's lymphoma, besides rare cases of metastatic transitional cell carcinoma of the bladder and Hodgkin lymphoma's)[5]
> - Less common causes (gout, monoclonal gammopathy, iron-deficiency anemia, and celiac disease)[5]

> **BOX 2: Clinical grade for prurigo nodularis.**
> - Mild: ≤20 cutaneous lesions
> - Moderate: 20–100 cutaneous lesions
> - Severe: >100 cutaneous lesions

According to Zeidler et al.,[3] clinical graduation for PN was proposed by Jasmin Pölkin in 2018, (unpublished data) as described in **Box 2**.

Our patient during the first consultation was classified as a case of a moderate grade of PN.

Epidemiologic data about the prevalence and incidence of PN is unfortunately lacking.[3] There are case series indicating that all age groups, including children, can be affected by PN.[3,7] However, the elderly were found to be the most frequently affected patient group[7,8] as well as observed in our patient.

The histopathological examination of nodular cutaneous lesions in PN under optic microscopy revealed increased dermal nerve fiber density and changes in many types of skin cells, including mast cells, Merkel cells, epidermal keratinocytes, dendritic cells (DCs), endothelial cells, and collagen fibers.[1] These cells cause inflammation and pruritus through the release of tryptase, interleukin-31 (IL-31), prostaglandins, eosinophil cationic protein, histamine, and other mediators such as neuropeptides, including substance P, calcitonin gene-related peptide (CGRP) and nerve growth factor (NGF).[1] Interestingly, cutaneous biopsies of patients with PN exhibit a 50-fold upregulation of IL-31 mRNA when compared with healthy skin biopsies.[9]

Immunological and genetic studies have delineated allergic inflammatory pathways common to several disorders such as AD, asthma, and food allergy, among others, and driving pathogenesis, key among which is the interleukin 4 receptor (IL-4R) pathway.[10] The IL-4/IL-13/IL-4R axis promotes T helper cells type 2 (Th2) differentiation, which mediates the pro-allergic adaptive immune response.[10] Once IL-4 or IL-13 binds to the receptors, it triggers the transphosphorylation and

Iking et al.[7] published a study about an etiological survey in a consecutive cohort of 108 patients suffering from prurigo. In their study, 36.1% were male, with mean age of 61.5 ± 16.7 years, and interestingly, nearly half (46.3%) of all PN patients had either an atopic predisposition or an AD as a single cause of PN (18.5%) or as one co-factor of PN of mixed origin (27.8%).[7] Then, several authors concluded that atopic predisposition is a major factor involved in nearly half of PN patients.[7]

activation of receptor subunit-associated Janus family protein kinases (JAKs), including JAK1, JAK3, and JAK2.[10]

Dupilumab is an IgG4 human monoclonal antibody (mAb) that binds IL-4Ra, inhibits IL-4R signaling induced by both IL-4 and IL-13, and downregulates Th2 inflammation in AD and other allergic diseases.[10] At the molecular level, Dupilumab therapy lowered the signature of >800 genes affected in AD, including Th2 chemokines, T-cell proliferation, and DC genes.[11] Dupilumab decreases in mRNA expression of genes related to epidermal hyperplasia (*K16* and *MKI67*), T cells, and DCs (CD1b and CD1c) and potent inhibition of Th2-associated chemokines (CCL17, CCL18, CCL22, and CCL26) were noted without significant modulation of TH1-associated genes (*IFNG*).[11] These actions may explain the good response of Dupilumab in the PN treatment.

Skin lesions of chronic AD include increased infiltration by T cells, DCs, and eosinophils;[10] this tissue inflammatory pattern is remarkably similar to that found in lesions of PN. Although AD has been classified as a Th2-dominated disease, other T-cell subsets (Th22, Th17, and Th1 cells) might also contribute to pathogenesis. As mentioned above, some authors found in PN, upregulation of IL-31 mRNA.[9] The binding of IL-31 to its receptors activates powerful signaling pathways (i.e., the activation of JAK1 and JAK2 and the start of the JAK-STAT pathway).[10]

Thus, IL-31 was regarded as a novel player in type 2 inflammation. This theory was supported by the discovery that Th2 cells are one of the main producers of IL-31, and there is a positive correlation between IL-31 and AD severity.[10]

IL-31 secretion depends on IL-4, but it is not only secreted by Th2 cells.[10] Also, other Th cell subsets that encounter IL-4 are able to release IL-31.[10] Moreover, elevated IL-31 levels contribute to specific symptoms such as itching, skin lesions, and localized irritation/inflammation of AD.[10]

In a study that investigated the mRNA levels and immunoreactivity of NGF, IL-31, thymic stromal lymphopoietin, and endothelin axes in both lesional and perilesional skin in PN, Zhong et al.[12] observed higher expression of IL-31 mRNA in lesions from the five atopic patients than in those from the six nonatopic patients. These results suggest a much more important role of IL-31 in atopic versus nonatopic PN patients.[12]

All these findings support the use of Dupilumab in PN. Also, when dupilumab was applied to our patient, it gave excellent result in the pruritus and eczema control.

Prurigo nodularis is an orphan disease and given the high pruritic and chronic nature of this condition, there is a very high burden of diseases related to this entity, including high rates of associated anxiety and depression among PN patients, besides the high impact on the quality of life (QOL).[5] Chronic pruritus also negatively impairs sleep as well as QOL.[5] Our patient noticed high anxiety and poor QOL due to chronic sleep loss related to pruritus and uncontrolled scratching. After the first month of Dupilumab therapy, the gain of values on the VAS for pruritus was 80% (10 to 2), and he noticed a better quality of sleep.

Zhai et al.[13] in a retrospective study enrolled 20 patients with chronic recalcitrant pruritus (9 PN; 5 uremic pruritus; 4 chronic idiopathic pruritus; 1 lichen planus, and 1 eosinophilic dermatosis related to hematologic malignancy) and demonstrated under off-label use of Dupilumab as a successful endpoint at reducing itch in all patients, leading to complete resolution in 12/20 patients and an overall mean of numeric rating scale itch intensity (NRSi) of 7.55. Dupilumab was well tolerated with no significant adverse effects, as occurred with our patient.

Among 90 AD adult patients [52 males (57.7%); mean age = 44.6 years; range = 18–66 years) treated with dupilumab by Napolitano et al.[6] in two Italian university hospitals (Napoli and Catanzano), in 9 (5 females and 4 males) (10.0%) of 90 cases, a generalized PN (GPN) was included and they were affected by one or more atopic comorbidities (allergic rhinitis, asthma, and allergic conjunctivitis). The total IgE serum level was above normal in all patients (mean = 1,555 kU/L; range = 657–2,269 kU/L). The nine GPN patients were treated with Dupilumab administered in the standard dosing regimen (600-mg induction dose and 300 mg every 2 weeks thereafter).[6] The evaluation of the results was made after 16 weeks of treatment. In all the patients, a marked clinical improvement was observed, confirmed by the significant improvement in Eczema Area and Severity Index (EASI; mean ± SD = 30.5 ± 5.68 at t0 vs. 8 ± 2.59 at t1, p < 0.001), Dermatology Life Quality Index (DLQI; mean ± SD = 18.6 ± 5.26 at t0 vs. 3 ± 2.34 at t1, p < 0.001), and pruritus VAS score (mean ± SD = 9.15 ± 0.88 at t0 vs. 2.75 ± 0.7 at t1, p < 0.001) values. No adverse events were reported. No patient dropped out.[6]

We are able to find 41 PN patients treated with Dupilumab in PubMed/Medline (January 2019 to March 2020) in off-label use. Our patient was the oldest (87-year-old male) reported until now. The second one was reported by Giura et al.[14] as a case report of an 85-year-old woman who had developed itch and nodular excoriated lesions in the last 3 years but without a history of atopic manifestations.

The therapeutic approach for PN is based on case series and clinical experience: corticosteroids, phototherapy (especially UVB-narrow band), topical immunomodulators (topical calcineurin inhibitors) and immuno-suppressant agents (cyclosporine, azathioprine, mycophenolate mofetil, and methotrexate),[14,15] and neuromodulators such as gabapentin and pregabalin,[15] thalidomide[15] that, however, have significant potential undesirable side effects, especially in elderly patients. Our patient had previously treated himself with oral and infiltrative corticosteroids, methotrexate, mirtazapine, and hydroxyzine and experimented several systemic adverse effects.

Current therapies for PN aim to suppress the itch-scratch cycle and include a myriad of topical agents, such as steroids, calcineurin inhibitors, and neuromodulators such as capsaicin.[15] Topical agents are frequently unsuccessful, and this aspect was experimented by our patient. Systemic agents are often needed, including intralesional steroids, antipruritic agents such as oral antihistamines, neuromodulators such as gabapentin and pregabalin, and phototherapy.[15,16] In more severe cases, immunosuppressive agents such as thalidomide, cyclosporine, mycophenolate mofetil, azathioprine, and methotrexate have been used with varying success and come with a host of undesirable side effects,[15,16] as observed in our patient. Another aspect of the systemic immunosuppressive use in tropical countries is the endemic infectious diseases, such as gastrointestinal parasitosis (prophylaxis of Strongyloidiasis is mandatory, as performed in our patient), and the risk of these patients during the elderly age to develop a severe infectious endemic diseases such as dengue/zika/chikungunya[17] or a new epidemic virus, such as the recent pandemic Coronavirus disease (COVID-19).[18]

In general, Dupilumab is well tolerated, with few serious adverse effects being reported.[19] Adverse effects can include nasopharyngitis, headache, conjunctivitis, and injection-site reactions.[19] In multiple clinical trials, patients on dupilumab had fewer skin infections compared to patients on placebo.[15] Other possible adverse events reported included a relationship between dupilumab administration and development of alcohol flushing in one case, transient skin erythema and peeling, local site reactions, herpes simplex infections, and alopecia.[19]

CONCLUSION

Although until now we treated this single elderly PN patient with dupilumab, this mAb was a safe, and efficacious therapy, especially with fast action in reducing severe pruritus. More double-blinded studies involving multicenter institutions who enroll PN patients should be encouraged to prove the efficacy and safety of Dupilumab applied to this orphan condition with a poor QOL.

KEY MESSAGES

- Prurigo nodularis is a recalcitrant chronic orphan dermatosis, and at least 50% of these patients present atopic diathesis.
- There is a poor QOL, anxiety, depression, and social isolation among patients with prurigo nodularis.
- Often, topical and systemic treatments are unable to control the itching and cutaneous lesions; besides, they may cause several adverse effects in these patients, especially in the elderly.
- Dupilumab treatment, although it impacts high economic costs from the health system in developing countries, might improve PN and offer the best quality of life for these PN patients.

REFERENCES

1. Zeidler C, Tsianakas A, Pereira M, Ständer H, Yosipovitch G, Ständer S. Chronic prurigo of nodular type: A review. Acta Derm Venereol. 2018;98:173-9.
2. Miyachi Y, Okamoto H, Furukawa F, Imamura S. Prurigo nodularis. A possible relationship to atopy. J Dermatol. 1980;7:281-3.
3. Zeidler C, Yosipovitch G, Ständer S. Prurigo nodularis and its management. Dermatol Clin. 2018;36:189-97.
4. Hyde JN. A Practical Treatise on Disease of the Skin for the use of Students and Practitioners, 1st edition. Philadelphia: Henry C. Lea's Son & Co.; 1883.
5. Kwon CD, Khanna R, Williams KA, Kwatra MM, Kwatra SG. Diagnostic workup and evaluation of patients with prurigo nodularis. Medicines (Basel). 2019;6:97.
6. Napolitano M, Fabbrocini G, Scalvenzi M, Nisticò SP, Dastoli S, Patruno C. Effectiveness of dupilumab for the treatment of generalized prurigo nodularis phenotype of adult atopic dermatitis. Dermatitis. 2020. doi: 10.1097/DER.0000000000000517. [Epub ahead of print].
7. Iking A, Grundmann S, Chatzigeorgakidis E, Phan NQ, Klein D, Ständer S. Prurigo as a symptom of atopic and non-atopic diseases: aetiological survey in a consecutive cohort of 108 patients. J Eur Acad Dermatol Venereol. 2013;27:550-7.
8. Amer A, Fischer H. Prurigo nodularis in a 9-year-old girl. Clin Pediatr (Phila). 2009;48:93-5.
9. Sonkoly E, Muller A, Lauerma AI, Pivarcsi A, Soto H, Kemeny L, et al. IL-31: a new link between T cells and pruritus in atopic skin inflammation. J Allergy Clin Immunol. 2006;117:411-7.
10. Harb H, Chatila TA. Mechanisms of dupilumab. Clin Exp Allergy. 2020;50:5-14.
11. Hamilton JD, Suárez-Fariñas M, Dhingra N, Cardinale I, Li X, Kostic A, et al. Dupilumab improves the molecular signature in skin of patients with moderate-to-severe atopic dermatitis. J Allergy Clin Immunol. 2014;134:1293-300.
12. Zhong W, Wu X, Zhang W, Zhang J, Chen X, Chen S, et al. Aberrant expression of histamine-independent pruritogenic mediators in keratinocytes may be involved in the pathogenesis of prurigo nodularis. Acta Derm Venereol. 2019;99:579-86.
13. Zhai LL, Savage KT, Qiu CC, Jin A, Valdes-Rodriguez R, Mollanazar NK. Chronic pruritus responding to dupilumab-a case series. Medicines (Basel). 2019;6:72.
14. Giura MT, Viola R, Fierro MT, Ribero S, Ortoncelli M. Efficacy of dupilumab in prurigo nodularis in elderly patient. Dermatol Ther. 2020;33:e13201.
15. Rambhia PH, Levitt JO. Recalcitrant prurigo nodularis treated successfully with dupilumab. JAAD Case Rep. 2019;5:471-3.
16. Wiznia LE, Callahan SW, Cohen DE, Orlow SJ. Rapid improvement of prurigo nodularis with cyclosporine treatment. J Am Acad Dermatol. 2018;78: 1209-11.
17. Subbiah A, Mahajan S, Yadav RK, Agarwal SK. Intravenous immunoglobulin therapy for dengue capillary leak syndrome in a renal allograft recipient. BMJ Case Rep. 2018 19;2018:bcr2018225225.
18. Rothan HA, Byrareddy SN. The epidemiology and pathogenesis of coronavirus disease (COVID-19) outbreak. J Autoimmun. 2020;109:102433.
19. Maloney NJ, Tegtmeyer K, Zhao J, Worswick S. Dupilumab in dermatology: Potential for uses beyond atopic dermatitis. J Drugs Dermatol. 2019;18:S1545961619P1053X.

CASE 4

Two Cases of Severe Adult-onset Atopic Dermatitis Responsive to Dupilumab

Justin Greiwe, Jonathan A Bernstein

CASE PRESENTATION 1

A 69-year-old male presented to the office with a new-onset rash that started 3 years ago. The rash is located primarily on hands but has spread to involve both the upper and the lower extremities. On examination, the rash is nonevanescent and pruritic. There is no evidence of dermatographism but only a severe eczematous dermatitis that covers the patient's arms, legs, and neck.

To relieve the itch, the patient has been using a bag of ice which helps but only transiently. The rash seems to worsen in the sun and humidity. His primary care doctor prescribed multiple courses of high-dose topical corticosteroids as well as corticosteroid injections which improved the skin rash but only temporarily. The patient is the Safety Director for a digital dish satellite company, but this involves mainly office work and no exposures to chemicals or other potential sensitizing or irritating agents. His hobby is making model airplanes made of balsa wood, wood glue, and epoxy resins. He has used epoxy resins and various other glues in the past. He recalls using epoxy resins at the time the rash started but has avoided these glues ever since. He has no history of latex allergy but uses nitrile gloves when building the planes. He was previously seen by a dermatologist who performed patch testing which showed sensitivities to bacitracin, neomycin, ethylenediamine, and colophony. Additional patch testing to balsa wood and plywood was negative as well. He had no history of childhood atopic dermatitis (AD) or other atopic conditions. He was ultimately referred to the Allergy Department for further workup and evaluation due to the refractory nature of his chronic dermatitis which now involved the torso, extremities, and face. The Investigator Global Assessment (IGA) scale for AD was 4 at that time. Personal care products were changed to fragrant-free, dye-free, chemical-free product lines and he was encouraged to apply a barrier cream as well as a moisturizing lotion twice a day on the face and instructed to avoid materials related to model airplanes for the next few weeks. He was instructed to avoid materials related to model airplanes for the next few weeks and was encouraged to use a barrier cream as well as a moisturizing lotion twice a day on the face. In addition, clobetasol cream 0.05% was prescribed to be applied to his hands and other involved regions once daily except the face. He was instructed to apply an occlusive dressing for 2 weeks over his hands and forearms along with a trial of Elidel 1% to involved areas of the face. The skin biopsy revealed parakeratosis, acanthosis, spongiosis, exocytosis, and a mild superficial lymphocytic infiltrate. The final biopsy diagnosis was subacute to chronic spongiotic dermatitis highly consistent with AD. Subsequent serologic testing to assess his allergic status revealed a total immunoglobulin E (IgE) 37 and serum-specific IgE (sIgE) slightly positive to dust mite. On his return visit 4 weeks later, he indicated that the topical therapies, good skin care, and avoidance were not effective. Based on clinical course and poor response to treatment, it was decided to start dupilumab 300 mg every 2 weeks after a 600-mg initial loading dose. Over the course of the next few months, his eczematous rash and pruritus improved significantly, especially over the face and hands. The patient also noted significant improvement in the quality of life stating: "I feel like I'm getting my life back together."

CASE PRESENTATION 2

A 60-year-old male with a history of allergic contact dermatitis (ACD), type 2 diabetes mellitus, obstructive sleep apnea, and chronic obstructive pulmonary disease presented for further evaluation for persistent eczema. Previous patch testing by the dermatologist was positive to Balsam of Peru, phenylenediamine, parabens, bacitracin, and neomycin. There had been no known exposures to products containing these chemicals. He had been treated with various high-potency topical corticosteroid ointments and creams with poor control. His total IgE level was >1,000 and specific IgE testing to aeroallergens was positive to dust mite only. In addition to aggressive moisturization and good skin care, he was treated with hydroxychloroquine and phototherapy with good response but was subsequently lost to follow-up. 3 years later, he returned with persistent pruritic eczematous dermatitis primarily involving his lower extremities. His physicians had attributed the severe itch and skin changes to the poor control of diabetes. Initially, treatment of the severe itch with gabapentin 600 mg twice daily was attempted in conjunction with aggressive moisturization and better diabetes control. This proved ineffective and the eczematous dermatitis worsened resulting in ulcerations of the lower extremities believed due to scratching. Other topical antiscabies agents and systemic therapies including Antistaphylococcal antibiotics, potent first-generation antihistamines, methotrexate, and UVA/UVB phototherapy were attempted without success. The only treatment that provided relief was high doses of oral corticosteroids which further contributed to poor diabetes control. Finally, a skin biopsy was performed that revealed evidence of spongiotic dermatitis. Laboratory testing revealed mild elevations in erythrocyte sedimentation rate (ESR) and C-reactive protein (CRP) but no evidence of peripheral eosinophilia. Despite adherence with all of the above treatments and avoidance of all contact allergens, the patient still required multiple courses of oral prednisone and antibiotics for superficial skin infections throughout the year. He required a daily low dose of prednisone between 5 and 10 mg a day to control the itching. A bone density test was obtained to assess for osteoporosis due to frequent corticosteroid use which showed evidence of osteopenia. The patient was started on vitamin D, calcium, and a bisphosphonate. Surprisingly, his glycated hemoglobin (HbA1C) remained stable. Given the refractory nature of his chronic eczematous dermatitis, a biopsy consistent with spongiotic dermatitis, and a high total IgE level it was felt that his diagnosis was consistent with adult-onset AD, and dupilumab 300 mg subcutaneously every 2 weeks after an initial 600-mg loading dose was initiated. After only a few months of treatment, the patient was able to taper off oral prednisone with clearing of his skin and healing of the skin ulcerations and has continued to do well.

DISCUSSION

Atopic dermatitis (AD) is a systemic chronic inflammatory disease characterized by eczematous lesions, intense pruritus, immune dysregulation, skin barrier dysfunction, and dysbiosis.[1] AD most commonly presents in childhood and 80–90% are diagnosed within the first 5 years of life. In children, the eczema typically involves the flexural surfaces of the elbows and knees as well as the head, neck, hands, and feet.[2] While most AD cases typically resolve by school age or puberty, some children with AD have chronic symptoms that persist into adulthood. Studies have estimated that approximately 25–30% of cases persist from childhood to adolescence or adulthood[3,4] with 7% of US adults affected by AD.[5] Of that 7%, one in four adults with AD reports adult onset of his/her disease.[6] Adult-onset AD seems to be associated with more heterogeneic skin manifestations and is believed to represent a distinct phenotype from the childhood-onset form of AD that deserves special consideration. Unlike childhood-onset AD which has been linked to barrier disruption and the atopic march, adult-onset AD is associated with lower rates of atopic disease (i.e., allergic rhinitis, conjunctivitis); distinct lesional distribution involving mainly the head, neck, and hands rather than flexural involvement; and increased prevalence of nummular eczematous lesions.[7] Despite their phenotypical differences, adult- and childhood-onset AD appear to have similar severity, symptomatology, and quality of life impairment and should be approached in a similar manner with regard to skin hygiene, moisturization, and barrier repair.[7]

Unlike childhood-onset AD, the mechanism of adult-onset AD remains unclear but likely involves various multiple genetic and immunologic pathways that are influenced by environmental determinants. Rupnik et al. investigated the influence of filaggrin gene (*FLG*) mutations on early- versus late-onset development of AD, ACD, and chronic irritant contact dermatitis in a cohort of 241 AD patients.[8] They identified that four of the most common *FLG* loss-of-function mutations were associated with the early-onset but not late-onset form of AD.[8]

Currently, adult-onset AD is diagnosed based on a combination of the clinical presentation, involved skin distribution, past medical history, and physical examination in addition to ruling out other conditions that could mimic AD. To date, there are no definitive gold standard diagnostic criteria for AD although various approaches have been proposed over the years. Hanifin and Rajka (HR) criteria are probably the most well known, but various iterations of these criteria have been subsequently proposed in Europe and Asia [United Kingdom Working Party's diagnostic criteria, Kang and Tian criteria, Reliable Estimation of Atopic dermatitis in ChildHood (REACH)] with no diagnostic criteria specifically for adult-onset AD. A summary of some of the diagnostic criteria currently available for diagnosing AD is given in **Box 1**.

A major obstacle in setting up standard diagnostic criteria for AD is the lack of definitive biomarkers as well as the heterogeneity of AD.

As the above cases demonstrate, a diagnosis of adult-onset AD can be very difficult to differentiate from other chronic dermatitis conditions including psoriasis which can delay the diagnosis. The differential diagnosis includes ACD, mycosis fungoides/cutaneous T-cell lymphoma (CTCL), psoriasis, and scabies. Patch testing should be performed to rule out ACD. Skin biopsy can rule out other causes such as psoriasis, but findings of spongiotic dermatitis are nonspecific.[8] Skin-prick testing or sIgE testing, total IgE, and an absolute eosinophil count can help discern adult- from childhood-onset AD as adult-onset AD exhibits lower rates of atopic disease.

Treatment for adult-onset AD should follow the same approaches recommended for childhood-onset AD with a step-care approach focusing on basic skin care and trigger avoidance in conjunction with low-medium-high potency topical corticosteroids, antiseptic measures, and nonsteroidal topical agents such as phosphodiesterase E4 and calcineurin

BOX 1: Various diagnostic criteria for atopic dermatitis.

1980: Hanifin and Rajka diagnostic criteria (requires 3 major + 3 minor)[9]

- *4 Major criteria*
  - Pruritus
  - Typical morphology and distribution
    - Flexural lichenification in adults
    - Facial and extensor eruptions in infants and children
  - Chronic or chronically relapsing dermatitis
  - Personal or family history of atopy
- *23 Minor criteria*
  - Xerosis
  - Ichthyosis/palmar hyperlinearity, keratosis pilaris
  - Immediate (type I) skin test reaction
  - Elevated serum IgE
  - Early age of onset
  - Tendency toward cutaneous infections, impaired cell-mediated immunity
  - Tendency toward nonspecific hand or foot dermatitis
  - Nipple eczema
  - Cheilitis
  - Recurrent conjunctivitis
  - Dennie–Morgan infraorbital fold
  - Keratoconus
  - Anterior subcapsular cataracts
  - Orbital darkening
  - Facial pallor, facial erythema
  - Pityriasis alba
  - Anterior neck folds
  - Itch when sweating
  - Intolerance to wool and lipid solvents
  - Perifollicular accentuation
  - Food intolerance
  - Course influenced by environmental and emotional factors
  - White dermographism, delayed blanch

1987: Kang and Tian diagnostic criteria (requires 1 basic + 3 minor)[10]

- *2 Basic features*
  - Chronic or chronically relapsing pruritic dermatitis
  - Personal or family history of atopy

Continued

Continued

- *6 Minor features*
  - Onset before 12 years of age
  - Xerosis, ichthyosis, or palmar hyperlinearity
  - Allergic conjunctivitis, food intolerance, immediate skin reactivity, eosinophilia, or elevated serum IgE level
  - Tendency to cutaneous infections or impaired cell-mediated immunity
  - Facial pallor, white dermatographism, or delayed blanch
  - Periorbital darkening, perifollicular accentuation, or tendency to nonspecific hand and foot dermatitis

1994: United Kingdom Working Party's diagnostic criteria (requires 1 major + 3 minor)[11]

- *1 Major criteria*
  - Individual must have an itchy skin condition
- *5 Minor criteria*
  - History of flexural involvement (antecubital or popliteal fossa, front of ankles, wrists, or neck)
  - Visible flexural dermatitis
  - Personal history of asthma or hay fever (or history of atopic disease in parents or siblings if the patient is younger than 4 years of age)
  - History of generalized dry skin in the last year
  - Onset of rash under the age of 2 years

2016: Reliable Estimation of Atopic dermatitis in ChildHood (REACH) diagnostic criteria (requires 2 major or 1 major + 4 minor)[12]

- *2 Major criteria (Is your child correspondent to the following questions?)*
  - Has your child had an itchy rash which was coming and going in the last 12 months?
  - Has the itchy rash been detected on folds of the elbows or behind the knees in the last 12 months?
  - Have you or your family (father, mother, brothers, or sisters) had symptoms of "atopic dermatitis" or "asthma" or "allergic rhinitis" before or been diagnosed as one of the diseases before?

Continued

Continued

- 9 Minor criteria (Have your child had the following skin symptoms in the last 12 months?)
  - Has your child intermittently felt an itchy sensation, or had wrinkles, or had darkening, around the eyes?
  - Has your child intermittently felt an itchy sensation, or had oozing, around the ears?
  - Has your child intermittently has chapped or had oozing, around the lips?
  - Has your child intermittently felt an itchy sensation, or had thickening, or had darkening, around the neck?
  - Has your child intermittently felt an itchy sensation, or had oozing, or had thickening, under the buttock?
  - Has your child intermittently felt an itchy sensation, or had oozing, around the wrist or ankle joints?
  - Has your child had unusually dry skin?
  - Has your child felt itchy when he (or she) was sweating?

inhibitors. If these approaches are not effective, more aggressive options can be considered including wet wraps, UVA/UVB phototherapy, systemic immunosuppressants (cyclosporine, methotrexate, mycophenolate mofetil, azathioprine, or daily oral corticosteroids), or dupilumab which is the only one of the aforementioned agents approved for the treatment of AD. Dupilumab is a fully human IgG4 monoclonal antibody that inhibits interleukin (IL-4) and IL-13 cytokines by binding to the IL-4Rα subunit shared by the IL-4 and IL-13 receptor complexes. Increases in IL-4 and IL-13 type 2 cytokines in AD lesions are integrally involved in the pathogenesis of AD by inhibiting epidermal cell differentiation and synthesis of lipids and antimicrobial peptides.[13] It is an option for those patients where previous treatments have failed. Because dupilumab has an excellent safety profile, it would be preferred over systemic immunosuppressants which have significant associated adverse effects and requirements for ongoing laboratory monitoring.

CONCLUSION

Adult-onset AD remains a poorly described and under-recognized condition leading to delays in diagnosis and poor quality of life with significant direct and indirect healthcare costs. More research into the underlying immunopathogenesis is required to discern relevant biologic pathways, diagnostic biomarkers, and effective treatment with biologics such as dupilumab.

KEY MESSAGES

- Adult-onset AD is associated with more clinical and cutaneous heterogeneity and may represent a distinct phenotype compared with childhood-onset AD.
- Compared to childhood-onset AD, adult-onset AD has a much lower rate of atopic disease.
- Adult-onset AD lesions more consistently involve the head, neck, and hands as opposed to the flexural involvement often seen in childhood-onset AD and more frequently manifest as nummular eczematous lesions.
- A new-onset eczematous rash in an adult should in the differential diagnosis conditions include ACD, mycosis fungoides/CTCL, psoriasis, and scabies.
- Severe, poorly controlled cases of adult-onset AD that fail to respond to standard therapy warrant consideration for long-term treatment regimens with biologics that target specific pathways such as IL-4/IL-13.

REFERENCES

1. Bjerre RD, Bandier J, Skov L, Engstrand L, Johansen JD. The role of the skin microbiome in atopic dermatitis: a systematic review. Br J Dermatol. 2017;177:1272-8.
2. Lyons JJ, Milner JD, Stone KD. Atopic dermatitis in children: clinical features, pathophysiology, and treatment. Immunol Allergy Clin North Am. 2015;35: 161-83.
3. Thorsteinsdottir S, Stokholm J, Thyssen JP, Nørgaard S, Thorsen J, Chawes BL, et al. Genetic, clinical, and environmental factors associated with persistent atopic dermatitis in childhood. JAMA Dermatol. 2019;155:50-7.
4. Garmhausen D, Hagemann T, Bieber T, Dimitriou I, Fimmers R, Diepgen T, et al. Characterization of different courses of atopic dermatitis in adolescent and adult patients. Allergy. 2013;68:498-506.
5. Vakharia PP, Silverberg JI. Adult-onset atopic dermatitis: Characteristics and management. Am J Clin Dermatol. 2019;20:771-9.
6. Lee HH, Patel KR, Singam V, Rastogi S, Silverberg JI. A systematic review and meta-analysis of the prevalence and phenotype of adult-onset atopic dermatitis. J Am Acad Dermatol. 2019;80:1526-32.
7. Silverberg JI, Vakharia PP, Chopra R, Sacotte R, Patel N, Immaneni S, et al. Phenotypical differences of childhood- and adult-onset atopic dermatitis. J Allergy Clin Immunol Pract. 2018;6:1306-12.
8. Rupnik H, Rijavec M, Korosec P. Filaggrin loss-of-function mutations are not associated with atopic dermatitis that develops in late childhood or adulthood. Br J Dermatol. 2015;172:455-61.
9. Hanifin JM, Rajka G. Diagnostic features of atopic dermatitis. Acta Derm Venereol Suppl. 1980;92:44-7.
10. Kang K, Tian R. Atopic dermatitis. An evaluation of clinical and laboratory findings. Int J Dermatol. 1987;26:27-32.
11. Williams HC, Burney PG, Hay RJ, Archer CB, Shipley MJ, Hunter JJ, et al. The UK working party's diagnostic criteria for atopic dermatitis. I. Derivation of a minimum set of discriminators for atopic dermatitis. Br J Dermatol. 1994;131:383-96.
12. Lee SC, Bae JM, Lee HJ, Kim HJ, Kim BS, Li K, et al. Korean Atopic Dermatitis Association's Atopic Dermatitis Criteria Group. Introduction of the reliable estimation of atopic dermatitis in childhood: Novel, diagnostic criteria for childhood atopic dermatitis. Allergy Asthma Immunol Res. 2016;8:230-8.
13. Boguniewicz M, Fonacier L, Guttman-Yassky E, Ong PY, Silverberg J, Farrar JR. Atopic dermatitis yardstick: practical recommendations for an evolving therapeutic landscape. Ann Allergy Asthma Immunol. 2018;120:10-22.

CASE 5

A Quality-of-life Game Changer: Treatment with Dupilumab in an Adult with Atopic Dermatitis

Line Brok Nørreslet, Yasemin Topal Yüksel, Tamara Theresia Lund, Tove Agner, Simon Francis Thomsen

CASE PRESENTATION

A 43-year-old man of Pakistani descent with a history of atopic dermatitis (AD) since early childhood was referred to the Department of Dermatology, Bispebjerg Hospital, Denmark. After disease-free years in adolescence, his eczema relapsed with severe flares as well as chronic symptoms during college. He had a history of type 1 allergies toward inhaled allergens and foods, no family atopy disposition, and was a nonsmoker. He was treated with moisturizers, topical corticosteroids, and calcineurin inhibitors, respectively, which were insufficient to clear his eczema. Systemic therapy with azathioprine was added, which he failed to respond to. Later, systemic treatment with methotrexate was started, but also with insufficient response. He lived with his parents and had a job at the airport including physically strenuous work with luggage handling, which often worsened his eczema and caused sick leave. Ultimately, job change was necessary, and he started working at a hotel as a receptionist and night porter. At that time his AD was aggravated; he had an Eczema Area and Severity Index (EASI) score[1] of 34.1 (severe), an itch intensity score of 8 based on a visual analogue scale (VAS) ranging from 0 (none) to 10 (worst itch), and a sleep impact score of 9 based on a VAS ranging from 0 (no sleep disturbance) to 10 (worst score). In the Dermatology Life Quality Index (DLQI),[2] he scored 16 points (very large effect on a patient's life). Blood samples showed a serum total immunoglobulin E (IgE) of 23,400 IU/mL in addition to increased lactate dehydrogenase (LDH; 247 U/L) and eosinophils (0.74×10^9/L). Few months earlier during a severe flare, he had an IgE of 39,000 IU/mL. He did not exhibit any symptoms of hyper IgE syndrome or other diseases typically causing high IgE values (parasitic diseases, aspergillosis, etc.). He was started on dupilumab, and 2 weeks after the first injection (600 mg subcutaneously) he experienced remission of his eczema symptoms. Three months after compliant treatment in regard to the standard regimen of 300 mg subcutaneous injections every 2 weeks, the patient had an EASI score of 4.5 (mild), itch score of 1, and sleep score of 0 (**Fig. 1**).

No side effects were reported. Steady improvements continued to occur, and 18 months later the EASI score was 1.5 (mild) and itch, sleep, and DLQI were 0 (no effect at all on a patient's life).

He returned to the job at the airport and had no sick leave due to AD. He moved to an apartment of his own, his social abilities improved, and the fact that the intense itch had stopped made it possible to do sports. The total serum IgE decreased continuously and was 4,780 IU/mL after 18 months (**Fig. 2**), and at this time also serum LDH (133 U/L) and eosinophils (0.24×10^9/L) were normalized.

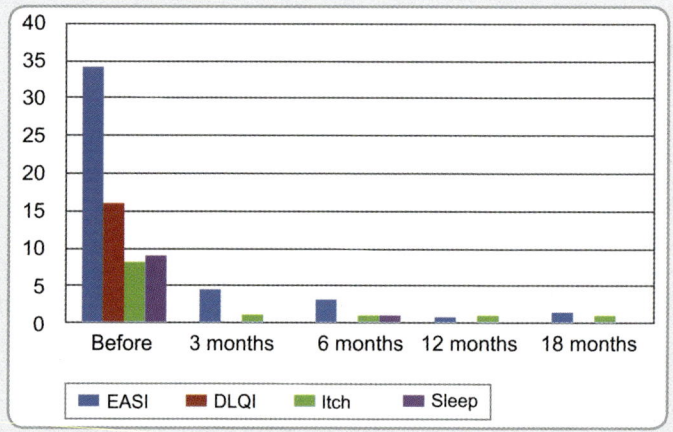

(DLQI: Dermatology Life Quality Index; EASI: Eczema Area and Severity Index)
FIG. 1: EASI, DLQI, itch and sleep score from baseline to 18 months later.

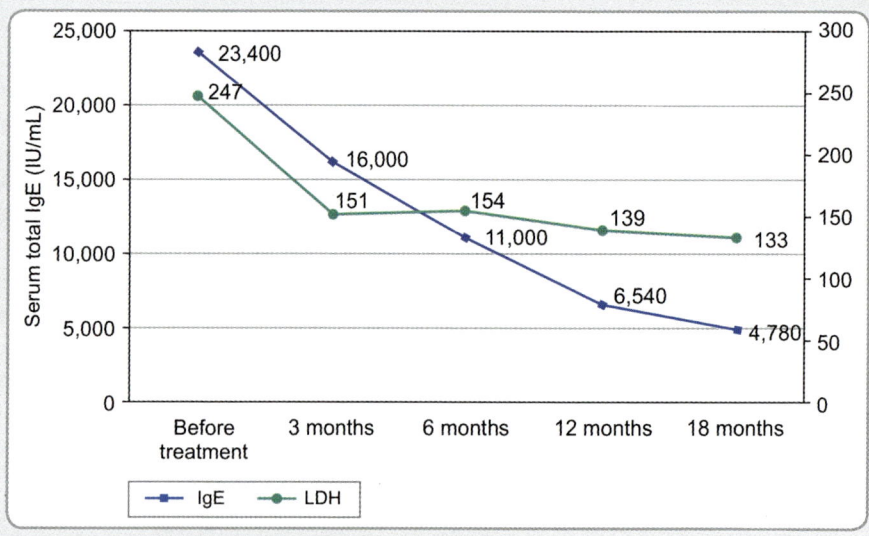

(IgE: immunoglobulin E; LDH: lactate dehydrogenase)
FIG. 2: Serum levels of IgE and LDH from baseline to 18 months later.

DISCUSSION

Atopic dermatitis (AD) is an inflammatory, enervating itchy disease with considerable negative impact on health-related quality of life (HR-QOL), comprising also the ability to interact in both social and work setting.[3] Today, inflammatory pathways in the pathogenesis of AD are described, and specific targeting may be superior to established immunosuppressive treatment approaches. New biological treatment options have shown efficacious results in adults with refractory AD. Dupilumab, a fully human IgG monoclonal antibody targeting the shared IL-4 and IL-13 receptor called IL-4Rα, was in 2017 the first FDA-approved biologic for moderate-to-severe AD.

We present a case of a male patient with severe AD since early childhood, and unusually high serum levels of IgE, whose HR-QOL and working ability increased dramatically after initiation of efficient treatment.

This case illustrates that efficient treatment of AD can lead to significantly improved HR-QOL. In our case, the patient had failed two previous systemic treatments and was started on dupilumab resulting in rapid and sustained improvements not only of pruritus and severity score, as previously reported, but also in social competences and working ability.[4-6]

In accordance with the literature, our case study exemplifies the significant impact that efficient treatment can have on HR-QOL, ability to work, and social relations for the individual.[1,7,8] Debilitating pruritus is a burden for patients with AD, causing profound negative psychosocial effects for the patients. Besides the HR-QOL advantages gained by efficient treatment as presented in our case, relief of anxiety and depression symptoms has been reported.[7]

Immunoglobulin E and LDH have been suggested as AD biomarkers correlating with both severity and treatment response[6,9] while others have not established this relationship.[8] Overall, a strong relationship between IgE and AD exists, but the functional pathomechanisms need clarification. About 80% of AD patients have elevated total serum levels of IgE,[10] which is to be expected as both IL-4 and IL-13 lead to increased IgE. Likewise, a significantly continuous reduction of serum IgE following dupilumab treatment is expected.[6,9] This was exemplified in our case, where the level of IgE was steadily reduced to one tenth of the original level after 18 months of treatment.

CONCLUSION

Severe AD can have a substantial, negative impact on HR-QOL for the affected individual. An efficient treatment should be sought, although it may be challenging and time consuming since several systemic treatments may have to be tried before an acceptable response is reached. New and emerging treatments, i.e., biologics and Janus kinase (JAK) inhibitors, expand the therapeutic repertoire. Symptom control is a relief for the patient and is rewarding also regarding HR-QOL, social aspects, and working ability.

KEY MESSAGES

- Severe atopic dermatitis negatively influences HR-QOL.
- Atopic dermatitis may cause increased sick leave and loss of job, which can however be reversed by effective treatment.
- Even very high serum IgE values are seen to decrease steadily after initiation of dupilumab.

REFERENCES

1. Hanifin JM, Thurston M, Omoto M, Cherill R, Tofte SJ, Graeber M. The eczema area and severity index (EASI): assessment of reliability in atopic dermatitis. EASI Evaluator Group. Exp Dermatol. 2001;10:11-8.
2. Finlay AY, Khan GK. Dermatology Life Quality Index (DLQI)—a simple practical measure for routine clinical use. Clin Exp Dermatol. 1994;19: 210-6.
3. Birdi G, Cooke R, Knibb RC. Impact of atopic dermatitis on quality of life in adults: a systematic review and meta-analysis. Int J Dermatol. 2020;59: e75-91.
4. Silverberg JI, Yosipovitch G, Simpson EL, Kim BS, Wu JJ, Eckert L, et al. Dupilumab treatment results in early and sustained improvements in itch in adolescents and adults with moderate-to-severe atopic dermatitis: analysis of the randomized phase 3 studies SOLO 1 and SOLO 2, AD ADOL, and CHRONOS. J Am Acad Dermatol. 2020;82(6): 1328-36.
5. Wang C, Kraus CN, Patel KG, Ganesan AK, Grando SA. Real-world experience of dupilumab treatment for atopic dermatitis in adults: a retrospective analysis of patients' records. I Int J Dermatol. 2020;59:253-6.
6. Olesen CM, Holm JG, Norreslet LB, Serup JV, Thomsen SF, Agner T. Treatment of atopic dermatitis with dupilumab: experience from a tertiary referral centre. J Eur Acad Dermatology and Venereol. 2019;33:1562-8.
7. Blauvelt A, de Bruin-Weller M, Gooderham M, Cather JC, Weisman J, Pariser D, et al. Long-term management of moderate-to-severe atopic dermatitis with dupilumab and concomitant topical corticosteroids (LIBERTY AD CHRONOS): a 1-year, randomised, double-blinded, placebo-controlled, phase 3 trial. Lancet (London, England). 2017;389:2287-303.
8. Ferrucci S, Casazza G, Angileri L, Tavecchio S, Germiniasi F, Berti E, et al. Clinical response and quality of life in patients with severe atopic dermatitis treated with dupilumab: A single-center real-life experience. J Clin Med. 2020;9
9. Jaworek AK, Szafraniec K, Jaworek M, Halubiec P, Wojas-Pelc A. The level of total immunoglobulin E as an indicator of disease grade in adults with severe atopic dermatitis. Pol Merkur Lekarski. 2019;47: 217-20.
10. Werfel T, Allam JP, Biedermann T, Eyerich K, Gilles S, Guttman-Yassky E, et al. Cellular and molecular immunologic mechanisms in patients with atopic dermatitis. J Allergy Clin Immunol. 2016;138:336-49.

CASE 6

Refractory Atopic Dermatitis in a Young Male Patient: Course and Symptoms Following Start of Dupilumab

Tamara Theresia Lund, Line Brok Nørreslet, Yasemin Topal Yüksel,
Tove Agner, Simon Francis Thomsen

CASE PRESENTATION

A 24-year-old male, Caucasian, and with atopic dermatitis (AD) since childhood, was in April 2017, referred to the outpatient clinic of the Department of Dermatology, Bispebjerg Hospital, for optimization of treatment. This patient presented himself with severely negatively impaired health-related quality of life (HR-QOL) due to AD in combination with a stressful work in the IT business, a busy social life, and several insufficient treatment attempts.

Prior treatment strategies on which the patient had failed included topical corticosteroid (TCS) group III, topical calcineurin inhibitors (TCIs), and immune-suppressive systemic treatment with azathioprine and methotrexate (MTX). Azathioprine did not have a sufficiently positive effect, and MTX was stopped after 6 weeks due to marked gastrointestinal side effects. Patch test was positive for lanolin, with no current relevance. Prick test was positive for dust, grass, animal hair, nuts, and apples.

At referral, approximately 50% of the skin was affected by AD with significant inflammation and scaling, almost erythrodermic. Eczema area and severity index (EASI)[1] score was 32.4 (severe AD). Severe itch was rated 8 by the patient on the Itch Numeric Rating Scale (itch NRS, scale 0–10 with 10 indicating worst symptoms) and impaired sleep was rated 5 by the patient on the scale for sleep disorder (sleep NRS, scale 0–10 with 10 indicating worst symptoms). Dermatology Life Quality Index (DLQI) was not registered at the first visit. High levels of immunoglobulin E (IgE) accompanied the symptoms (20,000 IU/L).

Treatment with cyclosporin (100 mg + 50 mg/day) was initiated after relevant preliminary tests, and although no side effects emerged, the treatment was discontinued after 4 months due to treatment failure with a continued clinically moderate-to-severe activity of AD. Biological treatment with dupilumab was started according to protocol with an initial dose of 600 mg subcutaneously followed by a maintenance dose of 300 mg subcutaneously every 2 weeks.

The patient responded as desired after 4 weeks with EASI dropping to 15.0, accompanied by decreasing levels of IgE (15,100 IU/L), but over the next months a further decrease in EASI, as would have been expected, was not seen. Concomitantly, all treatment with TCS had ceased. Regarding adverse events, the patient complained of conjunctivitis, which cleared when treated with antihistamine eyedrops. Subsequently, TCS for the body and TCI for the face were reintroduced on a daily basis and later as proactive treatment twice weekly. Two years later, the patient had cleared almost completely with EASI of 0.45, 0 on both NRS and sleep disorder scales, and IgE 1,160 IU/L resulting in a desired improvement in HR-QOL. The eczema continues to be under control, with a minimum of symptoms and no side effects from the treatment.

DISCUSSION

Often a lifelong companion, atopic dermatitis (AD) is a chronic skin disease not always easy to treat. The available treatment modalities span from emollient and TCS, avoidance of exacerbating factors in both personal and work life to immune-modulating and biological drugs.[2] HR-QOL may often be significantly affected in a negative direction and is an important factor, when deciding upon the treatment strategy. Insufficient disease control has been shown to be common among patients with moderate-to-severe AD, increasing the negative impact on HR-QOL.[3] Dupilumab, a new human anti-interleukin-4 receptor alpha monoclonal antibody, has shown to improve clinical signs, symptoms, and HR-QOL in AD patients where prior treatment strategies have failed.[4,5] This case presents the course of the disease in a young man with severe AD from admission to a dermatological department with severe AD and clearing of the disease.

Many factors influence the decision on which treatment a patient will benefit the most from. Not only severity of the disease, but also the patient's age, lifestyle, skin type, costs of treatment, side effects, individual preferences, and national treatment guidelines should be taken into consideration.

This case is an example of a young man with a lifelong history of recalcitrant AD. Stress from insufficient effect of various treatments affected the patient physically, impaired his ability to work, and led to a demotivating view on available treatment solutions.

Atopic dermatitis has been shown to have a noticeable negative impact on the patient's HR-QOL as well as being associated with depression and anxiety, which underlines the need for optimal treatment.[4,6] Today, patients with moderate-to-severe AD who have not benefitted from topical treatment, light therapy, or systemic treatment may be eligible for biological treatment.[5]

Dupilumab has been shown to efficiently treat AD in both phase-III trials and real life.[7,8] In the presented case, the patient responded well; however, after the initial improvement the patient stopped use of TCS and experienced flare-up of the disease and lack of further improvement. Cessation of TCS, used constantly or sporadically for years, will inevitably lead to flare-up and should not be mistaken for insufficient effect of treatment. Longer duration of treatment may also be required to reach the full effect of dupilumab in patients with severe AD as well as concomitant treatment with TCS has been shown to increase the effect of dupilumab.[9] Apart from a single incidence of conjunctivitis, which is a frequently reported side effect of dupilumab, no adverse events were reported.

CONCLUSION

Dupilumab may be considered in patients with moderate-to-severe AD. It is important to note that a rebound effect may occur when treatment with TCS has ceased. Treatment with dupilumab should in this case not be discontinued, but TCS should be reintroduced and tapered slowly, while sufficient effect of dupilumab should be waited for.

KEY MESSAGES

- Severe AD in young adults has significantly negative impact on HR-QOL.
- Consider treatment with biologics in case of severe refractory cases of adult AD and failure on other systemic treatments.
- Flare-up after 2–3 months of dupilumab treatment may be a consequence of stopping TCS and should not be seen as a side effect or lack of efficacy of dupilumab.

REFERENCES

1. Tofte S, Graeber M, Cherill R, Omoto M, Thurston M, Hanifin JM. Eczema area and severity index (EASI): A new tool to evaluate atopic dermatitis. J. Eur. Acad. Dermatology Venereol. 1998;11:S197.
2. Leung DYM, Bieber T. Atopic dermatitis. Lancet. 2003;361:151-60.
3. Simpson E, Guttman-Yassky E, Margolis D, Feldman S, Qureshi A, Hata T, et al. Association of inadequately controlled disease and disease severity with patient-reported disease burden in adults with atopic dermatitis. JAMA. 2018;154:903-12.
4. Maksimović N, Janković S, Marinković J, Sekulović LK, Živković Z, Spirić VT. Health-related quality of life in patients with atopic dermatitis. J. Dermatol. 2012;39:42-7.
5. Tsianakas A, Luger TA, Radin A. Dupilumab treatment improves quality of life in adult patients with moderate-to-severe atopic dermatitis: results from a randomized, placebo-controlled clinical trial. Br J Dermatol. 2018;178:406-14.
6. de Bruin-Weller M, Gadkari A, Auziere S, Simpson EL, Puig L, Barbarot S, et al. The patient-reported disease burden in adults with atopic dermatitis: a cross-sectional study in Europe and Canada. J Eur Acad Dermatol Venereol. 2020;34(5):1026-36.
7. Olesen CM, Holm JG, Nørreslet LB, Serup JV, Thomsen SF, Agner T. Treatment of atopic dermatitis with dupilumab: experience from a tertiary referral centre. J Eur Acad Dermatol Venereol. 2019;33:1562-8.
8. Simpson EL, Bieber T, Guttman-Yassky E, Beck LA, Blauvelt A, Cork MJ, et al. Two phase 3 trials of dupilumab versus placebo in atopic dermatitis. N Engl J Med. 2016;375:2335-48.
9. Blauvelt A, de Bruin-Weller M, Gooderham M, Cather JC, Weisman J, Pariser D, et al. Long-term management of moderate-to-severe atopic dermatitis with dupilumab and concomitant topical corticosteroids (LIBERTY AD CHRONOS): a 1-year , phase 3 trial. Lancet. 2020;389:2287-303.

CASE 7

Erythrodermic Early Onset Atopic Dermatitis Clinically Mimicking Mycoses Fungoides/Sezary Disease

Ferrucci S, Tavecchio S, Angilieri L, Germiniasi F, Berti E, Boneschi V

CASE PRESENTATION

A 58-year-old Caucasian man was suffering since his childhood of a classic early onset atopic dermatitis (AD) associated with allergic rhinoconjunctivitis and asthma due to multiple sensitization (mites, pollens). After skin improvement while teen, worsening of the flexural dermatitis took place in adulthood, up to episodes of suberythroderma characterized by wide areas of erythema, desquamation, crusting, and lichenification. For this situation, in the past, he underwent systemic therapy with courses of steroids and then with cyclosporine with some benefit for about 2 years; a short course with methotrexate was not tolerated.

Four years ago he was referred to our dermatologic department for a scaling erythemato-vesicular erythrodermic state, intensely itchy; shortly after, he started a new cycle of cyclosporine with good response except for hand and face.

Two years ago he was hospitalized in our clinic for another episode of erythroderma started shortly after the cyclosporine was stopped because of hypertension. To rule out the possibility of latent malignancies, in particular hematologic ones or cutaneous T-cell lymphoma, a number of investigations were performed: Chest X-ray, abdominal echography, complete blood cell count, lymphocyte subpopulations, and serum tumor markers. These exams resulted as normal except for hypereosinophilia (1.300/mm^3) and high immunoglobulins E level (3.100 kU/L). Furthermore, a lymph node ecography at laterocervical, axillae and groin was done detecting a reactive state. The skin biopsy revealed histopathology characteristics suggestive for mycosis fungoides (MF): small-to-medium lymphocytes with hyperchromatic and indented nuclei in small aggregates in the superficial and follicular epidermis along with a weak monoclonal T-cell receptor (TCR) gamma (Mix-B). However, clonal TCR-gamma rearrangement was not confirmed in a second skin biopsy; moreover, TCR-gamma was absent in peripheral blood and cytofluorimetry did not reveal aberrant CD4+ T-lymphocytes. On the basis that the diagnosis of MF/Sezary disease or other malignancies was ruled out and given the severity of his AD with Eczema Area and Severity Index (EASI) score of 48 and pruritus Numerical Rating Scale (NRS) score of 10, on November 2018, the patient started therapy with dupilumab: 600 mg subcutaneously on the first day followed by 300 mg every 2 weeks. The systemic steroid was rapidly tapered and at last suspended; only emollients to restore the cutaneous barrier and gentle detergents were allowed.

After 4 weeks from the beginning of the therapy he showed a good improvement of the dermatitis (EASI 18) and the itch (NRS 3), and his IgE level felt to 1,800 kU/L. After 16 weeks, he achieved further improvement with reduction of erythema and scaling and much less infiltration of the skin (EASI 10) associated with light itch (NRS 3) and further reduction of IgE level to 900 kU/L and eosinophilia to 7% (absolute count 600).

The patient was steadily improving along the next weeks until 60 weeks when EASI was 5 and itch NRS was 0. Sleep and Dermatology Life Quality Index (DLQI) also had an astonishing fall. Moreover, the patient's rhinoconjunctivitis and asthma were better in spring. It is of note that the only cutaneous sites not responsive to therapy are the face, in particular eyelids, and neck. Dupilumab was well tolerated by the patient without side effects.

Table 1 shows evaluated parameters at baseline and at 60 weeks.

TABLE 1: Evaluated parameters at baseline and week 60.

Dupilumab 300 mg every 2 weeks	EASI	PGA	Itch NRS	Sleep NRS	DLQI	Peripheral IgE kU/L—% eosinophils
Basal	43	4	10	8	12	3,100—12
60 weeks	5	0	0	0	1	290—7

(DLQI: Dermatology Life Quality Index; EASI: Eczema Area and Severity Index; NRS: Numerical Rating Scale; PGA: Physician Global Assessment)

DISCUSSION

Atopic dermatitis (AD) is a chronic inflammatory disease characterized by a complex pathophysiology that involves disruption of the skin barrier and type 2 immune response.[1] During the past years, significant therapeutic progress has been made in the field of the therapy of AD.[2] Dupilumab, a human monoclonal antibody that binds interleukin 4 (IL-4) receptor of the α subunit, is the first biologic agent targeting type 2 inflammation and is currently approved for the therapy of moderate-to-severe AD.[3,4]

We here report a paradigmatic case of severe early onset persistent AD. Partial or short response to usual therapies characterized the clinical course of the disease, for which several courses of systemic steroid and cyclosporine were employed. The prolonged immunosuppression during the years alerted us to perform investigations in order to rule out cutaneous and/or hemolymphatic malignancies before to treat the patient with dupilumab for AD. The shift to type 2 inflammation that takes place in AD patients could sometimes lead to clinical diagnosis of MF.[5] In fact, cutaneous histopathology initially suggested the latter diagnosis, subsequently not confirmed. Dupilumab has shown to switch off the upregulation of IL-4 and IL-13 and consequently the steadily inflammatory cutaneous state as well as the respiratory allergy.[6] It is not clear why some skin sites such as face, neck, or hand could have a limited good response to therapy or in some case worsen during it; perhaps the skin lifetime exposition to the environment (allergens, sun) in these areas favors a different cutaneous cytokines profile. Moreover, restoring the skin barrier with emollients has a strong impact on the course of AD because it seems to limit the transepidermal water loss and the prolonged immunological stimulation by allergens and chemicals through epidermal-derived cytokines.

KEY MESSAGES

- AD has different clinical presentations in adult patients and erythroderma has an important negative impact on the quality of life of the patients.
- The diagnosis of late-onset AD is clinical but frequently require examination to rule out other diagnoses.
- The therapy with dupilumab has proven to be effective, safe and manageable, with rapid improvement of pruritus, sleep, clinical manifestation, and quality of life of the patients. Moreover, the results persist over time.

REFERENCES

1. Fishbein AB, Silverberg JI, Wilson EJ, Ong PY. Update on atopic dermatitis: Diagnosis, severity assessment, and treatment selection. J Allergy Clin Immunol Pract. 2020;8(1):91-101.
2. de la O-Escamilla NO, Sidbury R. Atopic dermatitis: Update on Pathogenesis and therapy. Pediatr Ann. 2020;49:140-6.
3. De Wijs LEM, Bosma AL, Erler NS, Hollestein LM, Gerbens LAA, Middelkamp-Hup MA, et al. Effectiveness of dupilumab treatment in 95 patients with atopic dermatitis: daily practice data. Br J Dermatol. 2020;182:418-26.
4. Ferrucci S, Casazza G, Angileri L, Tavecchio S, Germiniasi F, Berti E, et al. Clinical response and quality of life in patients with severe atopic dermatitis treated with dupilumab: A single-center real-life experience. J Clin Med. 2020;9:E791.
5. Silvestre Salvador JF, Romero-Pérez D, Encabo-Durán B. Atopic Dermatitis in adults: A diagnostic challenge. J Investig Allergol Clin Immunol. 2017;27:78-88.
6. Licari A, Castagnoli R, Marseglia A, Olivero F, Votto M, Ciprandi G, et al. Dupilumab to treat type 2 inflammatory disease in children and adolescents. Paediatr Drugs. 2020. doi: 10. 1007/s40272-020-00387-2. [Epub ahead of print]

CASE 8

Food Allergy, Vaccination and Atopic Dermatitis Treatment in Children

Luis Felipe Ensina, Fernanda Sales da Cunha, Ana Paula Cusato-Ensina

CASE PRESENTATION

DAV is a 7-year-old male Caucasian patient, born and residing in São Paulo, Brazil. He has suggestive symptoms of atopic dermatitis (AD) since he was 6 months of age and visited our center for the first time at the age of 4 years.

At that time, his disease was poorly controlled, and quality of life was impaired by frequent eczema flares. He was taking high doses of hydroxyzine and chlorpheniramine daily, potent topical corticosteroids, topical calcineurin inhibitors, and over-the-counter skin lotions. He also had allergic rhinitis and asthma, treated and controlled with topical nasal steroids and salbutamol inhaler on demand.

Additionally, he had a history of neck and tongue itching and perioral redness minutes after eating 2 spoons of yogurt around 1 year before, with symptoms improving with desloratadine. Likewise, he had experienced mouth itching, vomiting, and diarrhea approximately 1 hour after eating an egg and had an alleged contact urticaria to cow's milk. Moreover, his mother complained about urticaria <12 hours after an influenza vaccine, with spontaneous recovery in 2 days, and worsening of the eczema and an asthma flare, a day after yellow fever vaccination (YFV).

Laboratory tests (ImmunoCAP) for serum allergen-specific immunoglobulin E (IgE) antibodies were performed: Egg white IgE 6.38 kU/L, egg yolk IgE 3.47 kU/L, ovomucoid IgE 5.01 kU/L, and cow's milk IgE 7.86 kU/L. Total IgE was 295 kU/L.

Egg and milk exclusion diet was recommended but had no impact in eczema severity. The soak and smear technique was initiated with some benefit, but the dermatitis went out of control during the subsequent months. The patient was experiencing sleep disorders because of pruritus during the night, deeply impacting his and his family's quality of life.

Treatment with cyclosporin was initiated, resulting in significant clinical improvement. He was able to sleep the whole night and his SCORing Atopic Dermatitis (SCORAD) score had a substantial drop. The combination of cyclosporin, topical corticosteroids, levocetirizine four-fold doses, and moisturizers was quite effective and, after 1 year of treatment, cyclosporin doses could be gradually reduced. Currently, symptoms are controlled with the association of an exclusion diet with proactive topical corticosteroids therapy, daily moisturizers, and on demand high doses of second-generation antihistamines.

DISCUSSION

Atopic dermatitis (AD) is a chronic, relapsing, inflammatory skin disease that occurs more commonly in children, but can also affect adults and has an age-specific typical morphology and distribution. It is a heterogeneous and multifactorial inflammatory skin disease, which can significantly impact the patient's quality of life.[1] In this discussion, we would like to not only stress the role of food allergy in AD, but also comment about antihistamines and cyclosporin treatment.

Food allergy has been well documented in approximately one-third of children with moderate-to-severe AD. The most common food allergies in patients with AD are milk, egg, and peanuts. Though sensitization classically occurs through the gastrointestinal tract, because of a gut barrier dysfunction and facilitated absorption of food protein, it has been shown that sensitization can also be achieved before ingestion through inflamed skin. A dysfunctional epidermal barrier may lead to the entry of various environmental triggers, such as food allergens, with subsequent percutaneous sensitization leading to the development of food allergy. Milk-based skincare products, for instance, might sensitize patients for milk protein and lead in the future to a food allergy.[2]

Accurate diagnosis of food allergy in AD patients is not easy to be done. It should take into consideration a good clinical history, laboratory tests, elimination diet if indicated, and even an oral food challenge, if necessary, to exclude or confirm a possible diagnosis.[3] Laboratory workup, therefore, should only be done in children with a clinical history of immediate reaction to a single food or in patients with a moderate-to-severe AD despite optimal skincare and currently ingesting a potential culprit food, which could actively contribute to worsening the eczema.[2] Extensive allergy workup should never be done and laboratory tests should be focused on specific food allergens, guided by clinical history. Clinicians must appreciate that a positive food-specific IgE test only denotes sensitization and may not confirm an allergy. Clinical history is key to the correct management of these patients.[3]

Taking into consideration all the vaccines that contain egg protein [Measles, Mumps, and Rubella (MMR), rabies, influenza and yellow fever], MMR and rabies vaccines have an insignificant amount of egg protein, and no special precautions need to be followed for egg-allergic patients receiving these vaccines. Yellow fever and influenza vaccines, however, have an amount of egg protein that is not neglectable.[3,4] Most influenza vaccines hold a very small amount of egg protein, which varies among manufacturers. Recent studies have shown that even individuals with confirmed egg allergy can safely receive the flu vaccine. No special precautions are needed for the administration of influenza vaccine to egg-allergic patients; it does not matter how severe the allergy reaction was.[4,5]

Yellow fever vaccine is broadly recommended in endemic areas, such as Brazil. The disease remains a public health problem and immunization is the most effective protective measure against it. A single dose provides lifelong immunity against yellow fever. The benefit of vaccination outweighs possible side effects or hypersensitivity reactions to the vaccine. Literature shows that patients with mild-to-moderate allergies to egg protein can undergo normal yellow fever vaccination supervised by physicians at a controlled site. The ones with an anaphylactic history to egg protein should undergo a desensitization protocol.[4]

First-generation sedating H1-antihistamines have been used in AD to promote sleep and reduce nocturnal scratching due to their sedative effects, despite the questionable involvement of histamine in AD pruritus. However, sedating antihistamines reduce the rapid-eye-movement (REM) sleep, affecting the quality of sleep, interfering directly in work efficiency in adults and learning skills in children. Differently, second-generation H1-antihistamines have shown to be safe even in high doses and for long periods, supporting their use in children and adults with AD.[6,7] Nevertheless, their effects markedly differ among patients and must be evaluated individually.[8]

Cyclosporine is considered to be the first-line option for patients with severe disease who require systemic immunosuppressive treatment and its duration should be guided by clinical efficacy and tolerance of the drug. Its improvement rate after 6–8 weeks' treatment is around 55%, but its side-effects profile may limit the long-term use.[6] However, although its relapse rate varies, it is suggested that the longer the treatment, the lower the chance of relapse.[9] Thus, a course of cyclosporine may be useful to improve the disease, which can be controlled only with topical therapy subsequently.

CONCLUSION

Food allergy should not be investigated in all AD patients but must be remembered in the moderate-to-severe cases, which have a clear cause–effect relationship with a food culprit. Even high-risk patients should undergo vaccination. Treatment should be individualized and aims both safety and long-term symptom control.

KEY MESSAGES

- Food allergy must be remembered in the moderate-to-severe cases of AD suggesting a cause–effect relationship with a food culprit.
- Treatment should be individualized with objectives of long-term symptom control and safety considerations.

REFERENCES

1. Fishbein AB, Silverberg JI, Wilson EJ, Ong PY. Update on atopic dermatitis: Diagnosis, severity assessment, and treatment selection. J Allergy Clin Immunol Pract. 2020;8:91-101.
2. Bergmann MM, Caubet J-C, Boguniewicz M, Eigenmann PA. Evaluation of food allergy in patients with atopic dermatitis. J Allergy Clin Immunol Pract. 2013;1:22-8.
3. Burks AW, Tang M, Sicherer S, Muraro A, Eigenmann PA, Ebisawa M, et al. ICON: Food allergy. J Allergy Clin Immunol. 2012;129:906-20.
4. Marinho AKBB, Ouricuri AL, Valente CFC, Fernandes FR, Saciloto G, Diniz L de C, et al. (2017). Vacina contra a febre amarela: reações adversas e populações de risco. Arquivos de Asma, Alergia e Imunologia. [online] Available from http://www.gnresearch.org/doi/10.5935/2526-5393.20170035 [Last accessed October, 2020].
5. Greenhawt M, Turner PJ, Kelso JM. Administration of influenza vaccines to egg allergic recipients: A practice parameter update 2017. Ann Allergy Asthma Immunol. 2018;120:49.
6. Wollenberg A, Barbarot S, Bieber T, Christen-Zaech S, Deleuran M, Fink-Wagner A, et al. Consensus-based European guidelines for treatment of atopic eczema (atopic dermatitis) in adults and children: Part II. J Eur Acad Dermatol Venereol. 2018;32:850-78.
7. Church MK, Maurer M. H1-Antihistamines and itch in atopic dermatitis. Exp Dermatol. 2015;24:332-3.
8. Saeki H, Nakahara T, Tanaka A, Kabashima K, Sugaya M, Murota H, et al. Clinical practice guidelines for the management of atopic dermatitis. J Dermatol. 2016;43:1117-45.
9. Sibbald C, Pope E, Ho N, Weinstein M. Retrospective review of relapse after systemic cyclosporine in children with atopic dermatitis. Pediatr Dermatol. 2015;32:36-40.

CASE 9

Do Not Miss Contact Allergy in Atopic Dermatitis Patients

Esra Saraç, Emek Kocatürk

CASE PRESENTATION

An 18-year-old female patient presented with itching and rash on the face and hand eczema. She had hand eczema since childhood, but it got worse since 2 years. The rash on the face started 6 weeks ago. She has been having dry skin, hand eczema, and itchy lesions on the flexural lesions since her childhood. She also had allergic rhinitis with a positive prick testing to house dust mites. She did not have a family history of atopic dermatitis (AD). She has started to work in a hairdresser saloon since 2 years. She noticed that her hand eczema worsened since she started working in the saloon. Her face started itching 6 weeks ago and then it became red and scaly. She denied use of any new cosmetic products on the skin. She recalls that her symptoms worsened after procedures of hair coloring and waxing.

Physical examination revealed desquamation and erythema on the face which was prominent at the periorbital region (**Fig. 1**), hyperkeratotic plaques and xerosis on the hands that were attenuated on the joints (**Fig. 2**), erythematous and scaly patches on both antecubital regions and popliteal fossa (**Fig. 3**), and generalized dryness of the skin and keratosis pilaris on the upper extensor arms (**Table 1**).

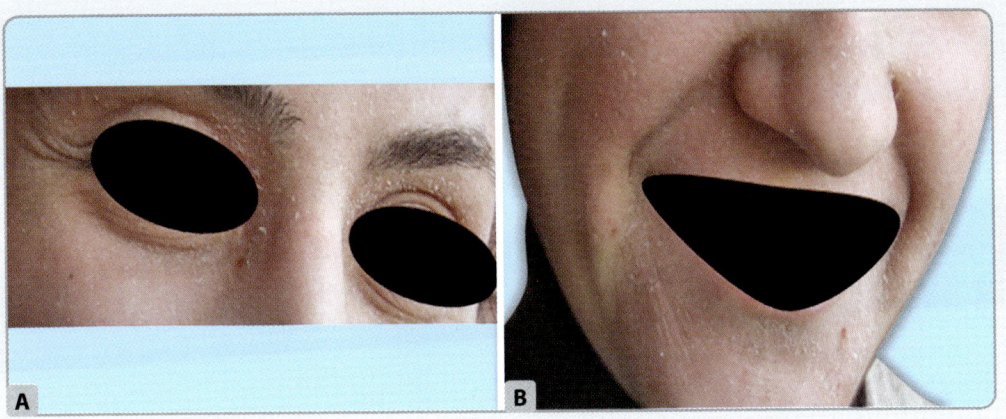

FIGS. 1A AND B: Desquamation and erythema on the face which was prominent in the periorbital region.

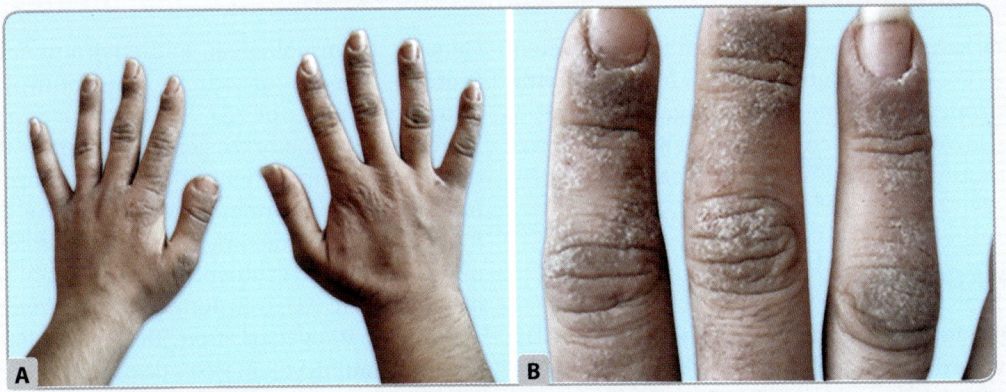

FIGS. 2A AND B: Hyperkeratotic plaques and xerosis on the hands that were attenuated on the joints.

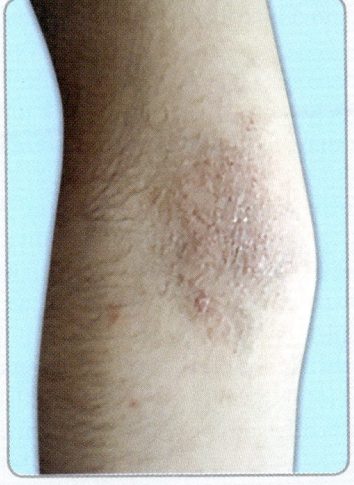

FIG. 3: Erythematous and scaly patches on the antecubital region.

TABLE 1:	Physical examination.
Lesion	**Comment**
Erythematous and desquamated patches on the antecubital and popliteal fossae	Related to atopic dermatitis
Generalized dryness of the skin	Related to atopic dermatitis
New developed erythema and desquamation on the face	Possible allergic contact dermatitis
Worsening of hand eczema presented with hyperkeratotic plaques, especially on the interphalangeal surfaces	Possible allergic contact dermatitis

INVESTIGATIONS

The serum IgE level was found to be elevated (1,134 IU/mL; **Table 2**). Patch testing with European Baseline Series (**Fig. 4**) showed a positive reaction to colophony and a positive reaction to paraphenylenediamine (PPD; **Table 2**).

DIAGNOSIS

Diagnosis of allergic contact dermatitis (ACD) over existing atopic dermatitis (AD) was made based on clinical clues, i.e., formation of eczematous lesions in new locations and worsening of previously existing lesions and occurrence of new lesions after starting work in a high-risk occupation.

Relevance of positive patch test reactions:
- Colophony: An allergen that may be found in epilating waxes.
- PPD: An allergen widely known to exist in hair dyes.
- The patient reports worsening of the symptoms after hair coloring and waxing.

The patient is treated with topical mometasone furoate cream and oral cetirizine tablet and advised to wear protective clothing while working. Change of occupation is advised for future.

DISCUSSION

Genetic, immunological, and environmental factors are involved in the complex etiopathogenesis of AD.[1] Although it is not known what exactly triggers the onset of the disease, the impairment of epidermal barrier function and immune dysregulation are the most highlighted factors; revealing the role of new T helper (Th) subtypes and the functions of cytokines in AD, transformed the hypothesis about etiopathogenesis from Th1/Th2 biphasic disease to multicytokine axes disorder.[2]

As it is known that the clinical presentation of AD differs according to the patient's age, it often effects the hands, feet, eyelids, head, and neck in adults in addition to flexural areas. The remarkable point in considering ACD or our patient presented here was the appearance of facial dermatitis which also involved the eyelids and recurrent hand dermatitis worsening in the workplace.

Distinct from AD, ACD is a type IV hypersensitivity reaction to a suspected allergen. The sensitizing potency of the allergen; the extent, frequency, and duration of the exposure; and local trauma or irritation influence the risk of contact sensitization.[3]

The coexistence of AD and ACD is controversial. Unlike the historical viewpoints suggesting less contact sensitivity in AD,[4-6]

TABLE 2:	Laboratory findings.	
Test	Result	Comment
Serum IgE level	1,134 IU/mL	Elevated/atopic dermatitis
Patch test	Colophony positive	Allergic contact dermatitis
Patch test	Paraphenylenediamine positive	Allergic contact dermatitis

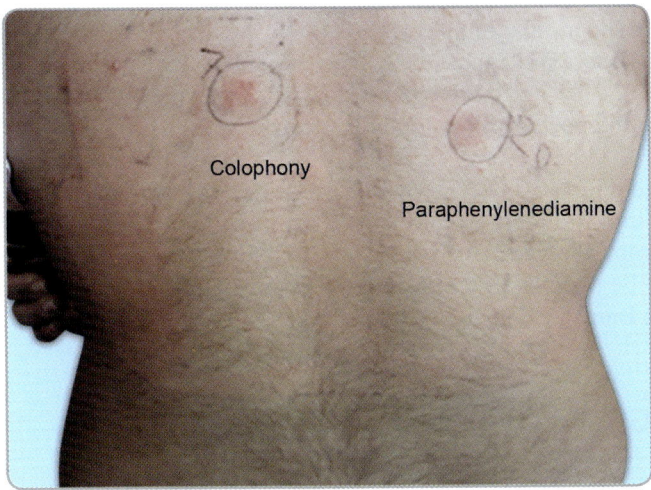

FIG. 4: Positive patch test reactions to colophony and paraphenylenediamine.

more recent studies highlight the increased risk of developing ACD.[3,7]

One of the theories elucidating this is the possible antigenic exposure from damaged skin barrier. Epidermal allergen penetration is increased in AD patients by virtue of skin barrier abnormalities including gene mutations, inflammation, and excoriations.[3,8] Environmental exposure to pollution, dust, and chemicals may contribute to a more defective epidermal barrier, adding to increased risk of allergen penetration.[9]

Another possible facilitator of contact sensitization may be the altered bacterial colonization of the atopic skin. It is shown in animal models that microbe-related substances can promote sensitization via stimulating the innate immune system.[10,11]

Besides, topical skin care products that are commonly used in the management of every AD stage are known to contain contact sensitizers.[12-14]

Performing patch test in AD should be considered in some circumstances recommended as (1) therapy-resistant or fast recurrent dermatitis, (2) atypically located dermatitis suggesting contact dermatitis (hand/foot, eyelid, head/neck, perioral), (3) refractory hand dermatitis in the working population, (4) AD that started after childhood, and (5) before starting systemic immunosuppressive therapy for AD.[15]

It should be kept in mind that irritant reactions can be more common in patients with AD.[16] Therefore, interpretation of the patch test could be difficult. Also, some medications given for AD may affect the accuracy of the patch test depending on the dosage and length of the therapy. Patch test is not recommended in situations such as taking daily systemic prednisone >10 mg or cyclosporine >2 mg/kg, intramuscular triamcinolone injection in the last 4 weeks, and topical steroid use on the patch testing area in the last 1 week.[15]

Patients with AD are more prone to have occupational skin diseases.[17] Working in high-risk occupation groups including hairdressers may affect the patient's quality of life and work performance. Previous studies in hairdressers have shown that the risk of developing contact dermatitis and contact sensitization increases after starting working.[18,19]

The top three occupationally related allergens in hairdressers are reported to be nickel sulfate, PPD, and glyceryl thioglycolate.[20] The patch test resulted positive for colophony and PPD in our patient.

Paraphenylenediamine is a very well-known allergen found in hair dyes, but colophony is not a common allergen in hairdressers. It was reported to be positive in 6 out of 399 hairdressers in the Danish Contact Dermatitis Group's study.[21] We suspect the source of colophony sensitization to be the waxing product in our patient. There are similar reports accusing epilating products as a source of colophony allergy in beauticians.[22]

CONCLUSION

The possible emergence of ACD should be considered in cases with AD, especially in patients working in high-risk occupations, and patch testing should be carried out for the proper management of these patients. An important point to be emphasized is that career guidance for individuals with AD is essential for preventing the occurrence of occupational eczema in high-risk occupations.

KEY MESSAGES

- ACD should be considered in cases with AD, especially in patients working in high-risk occupations.
- Patch testing should be carried out for the proper management of these patients.
- Career guidance for individuals with AD is essential for preventing the occurrence of occupational eczema in high-risk occupations.

REFERENCES

1. Boguniewicz M, Leung DY. Atopic dermatitis: A disease of altered skin barrier and immune dysregulation. Immunol Rev. 2011;241:233-46.
2. Malik K, Heitmiller KD, Czarnowicki T. An update on the pathophysiology of atopic dermatitis. Dermatol Clin. 2017;35:317-26.
3. Thyssen JP, McFadden JP, Kimber I. The multiple factors affecting the association between atopic dermatitis and contact sensitization. Allergy. 2014;69: 28-36.
4. Uehara M, Sawai T. A longitudinal study of contact sensitivity in patients with atopic dermatitis. Arch Dermatol. 1989;125:366-8.
5. Uehara M, Ofuji S. Patch test reactions to human dander in atopic dermatitis. Arch Dermatol. 1976;112: 951-4.
6. Jones HE, Lewis CW, McMarlin SL. Allergic contact sensitivity in atopic dermatitis. Arch Dermatol. 1973;107:217-22.
7. Halling-Overgaard AS, Kezic S, Jakasa I, Engebretsen KA, Maibach H, Thyssen JP. Skin absorption through atopic dermatitis skin: a systematic review. Br J Dermatol. 2017;177:84-106.
8. Jakasa I, Verberk MM, Esposito M, Bos JD, Kezic S. Altered penetration of polyethylene glycols into uninvolved skin of atopic dermatitis patients. J Invest Dermatol. 2007;127:129-34.
9. Kantor R, Silverberg JI. Environmental risk factors and their role in the management of atopic dermatitis. Expert Rev Clin Immunol. 2017;13:15-26.
10. Huang L, Kinbara M, Funayama H, Takada H, Sugawara S, Endo Y. The elicitation step of nickel allergy is promoted in mice by microbe-related substances, including some from oral bacteria. Int Immunopharmacol. 2011;11:1916-24.

11. Takahashi H, Kinbara M, Sato N, Sasaki K, Sugawara S, Endo Y. Nickel allergy-promoting effects of microbial or inflammatory substances at the sensitization step in mice. Int Immunopharmacol. 2011;11:1534-40.
12. Lubbes S, Rustemeyer T, Sillevis Smitt JH, Schuttelaar ML, Middelkamp-Hup MA. Contact sensitization in Dutch children and adolescents with and without atopic dermatitis - a retrospective analysis. Contact Dermatitis. 2017;76:151-9.
13. Hamann CR, Bernard S, Hamann D, Hansen R, Thyssen JP. Is there a risk using hypoallergenic cosmetic pediatric products in the United States? J Allergy Clin Immunol. 2015;135:1070-1.
14. Mailhol C, Lauwers-Cances V, Rance F, Paul C, Giordano-Labadie F. Prevalence and risk factors for allergic contact dermatitis to topical treatment in atopic dermatitis: a study in 641 children. Allergy. 2009;64:801-6.
15. Chen JK, Jacob SE, Nedorost ST, Hanifin JM, Simpson EL, Boguniewicz M, et al. A pragmatic approach to patch testing atopic dermatitis patients: clinical recommendations based on expert consensus opinion. Dermatitis. 2016;27:186-92.
16. Nassif A, Chan SC, Storrs FJ, Hanifin JM. Abnormal skin irritancy in atopic dermatitis and in atopy without dermatitis. Arch Dermatol. 1994;130:1402-7.
17. Drucker AM, Wang AR, Li WQ, Sevetson E, Block JK, Qureshi AA. The burden of atopic dermatitis: Summary of a report for the National Eczema Association. J Invest Dermatol. 2017;137:26-30.
18. Valks R, Conde-Salazar L, Malfeito J, Ledo S. Contact dermatitis in hairdressers, 10 years later: Patch-test results in 300 hairdressers (1994 to 2003) and comparison with previous study. Dermatitis. 2005;16:28-31.
19. Smith HR, Armstrong DK, Holloway D, Whittam L, Basketter DA, McFadden JP. Skin irritation thresholds in hairdressers: implications for the development of hand dermatitis. Br J Dermatol. 2002;146:849-52.
20. Warshaw EM, Wang MZ, Mathias CG, Maibach HI, Belsito DV, Zug KA, et al. Occupational contact dermatitis in hairdressers/cosmetologists: retrospective analysis of North American Contact Dermatitis Group data, 1994 to 2010. Dermatitis. 2012;23:258-68.
21. Schwensen JF, Johansen JD, Veien NK, Funding AT, Avnstorp C, Osterballe M, et al. Occupational contact dermatitis in hairdressers: an analysis of patch test data from the Danish contact dermatitis group 2002-2011. Contact Dermatitis. 2014;70:233-7.
22. Pesonen M, Suuronen K, Suomela S, Aalto-Korte K. Occupational allergic contact dermatitis caused by colophonium. Contact Dermatitis. 2019;80:9-17.

CASE 10

Successful Treatment of Epidermolysis Bullosa Pruriginosa with Anti-IgE Therapy (Omalizumab): A Case Report and 4 Years Follow-up

Salma Ahmed Taha, Maryam Ali Al-Nesf, Amina Mohamednoor Al-Obaidli

CASE PRESENTATION

A 34-year-old woman presented to the dermatology clinic with a 1-year history of pruritic bullous lesions after minor trauma to the skin. She had a past history of a resected thyroid papillary carcinoma and no childhood atopic disease. Her aunt and a maternal cousin also had bullous skin lesions. On examination, lichenoid papules were noted with a few vesicles, along with blisters on the extensor surfaces of upper and lower limbs, sparing nail, scalp, and mucous membranes (**Fig. 1**).

A punch skin biopsy revealed a subepidermal blister with a viable roof, epidermal and upper dermal edema, and perivascular lymphocytic, neutrophilic, and eosinophilic infiltrates. Immunofluorescent assays for immunoglobulin A (IgA), IgG, IgM, C1q, and C3 as well as serum epidermal IgG, celiac disease antibodies, and autoimmune workups were negative. Systemic glucocorticoids at a concentration of 0.5 mg/kg, along with cyclosporine and dapsone, failed to control her symptoms. Repeated skin biopsies were inconclusive. Serum total IgE increased to 2,587 kU/L (357 kU/L at baseline). Specific IgE titers for the dermatophagoides pteronyssinus and farinae were 2.23 and 5.08 kU/L, respectively. Whole exome sequencing (XomeDxPlus, NY, USA) showed a G2481D variant homozygous, nonconservative amino acid substitution mutation in the *COL7A1* gene. This variant has not been identified in the literature as a pathogenic or benign polymorphism; however, in silico analysis predicted a protein-damaging role. As her parent's DNA samples were not analyzed, a novel mutation could not be confirmed.

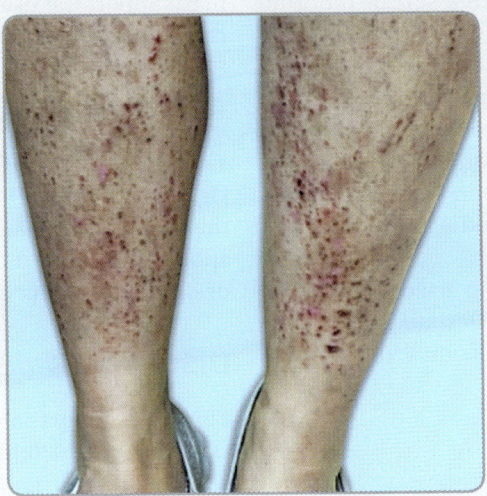

FIG. 1: Epidermolysis bullosa pruriginosa skin lesions (lichenoid papules with few vesicles and sloughed bullae seen on the patient's lower limbs).

DISCUSSION

Dystrophic epidermolysis bullosa (DEB) is caused by point genetic mutations in the *COL7A1* gene, which encodes the anchoring fibrils of the basement membrane to the underlying dermis; this mutation causes skin fragility and renders it more susceptible to friction.[1]

Epidermolysis bullosa pruriginosa (EBP) (OMIM #604129) is one of DEB's rare clinical phenotypes. Intractable pruritus and prurigo-like lichenified nodules are cardinal features of the adult disease form. Pruritus usually precedes or coexists with the severe clinical phenotype.[2] Identical *COL7A1* gene mutations could cause DEB or EBP clinical phenotype,[3] which suggests an additional unknown immunological or environmental mechanism. Rarity of the disease, a variable age of onset, and clinicohistological resemblance to other skin conditions make the diagnosis challenging.[4] Treatment options are limited to a few medications with a high side-effect burden making the treatment of pruritus even more difficult.[5]

Self-antigens instigating IgE-mediated autoimmune diseases were recently described.[5] Bullous pemphigoid (BP) was among the first of the autoimmune skin diseases demonstrating IgE's self-reactive role. The presence of autoreactive IgE antibodies against transmembrane protein BP180 and intracellular protein BP230 and IgE-coated mast cells in perilesional skin with BP180 peptides on these mast cells[6] supports the involvement of IgE autoantibodies in the pathogenesis of BP. Increased concentrations of serum and intralesion IgE were repeatedly observed in EBP cases;[2,7,8] however, a link to disease pathogenicity has not been established yet. Severe itching, which is central to a diagnosis of EBP, in the context of increased IgE suggests a causative role of IgE, particularly when skin lesions are provoked or increased by pruritus. Histamine which is a well-known pruritogen is released primarily by mast cells, when an allergen binds to the IgE receptor on their surface.[9] Autoreactive IgE has recently been identified in epidermolysis bullosa acquisita, which was previously viewed as a disorder reminiscent of DEB.[10] Similarly in EBP, autoimmune IgE could be the potential culprit triggering the inflammatory cascade in those who are genetically susceptible.

Omalizumab blocks free serum IgE from binding to the high-affinity FcεRI on mast cells. It has been licensed for treatment of chronic spontaneous urticaria (CSU), and postulated mechanisms include reducing the activity of IgG autoantibodies against FcεRI, reducing the activity of autoreactive IgE against unknown antigens, and reducing intrinsically abnormal IgE.[11]

Omalizumab has been used to treat BP successfully in the past.[12] Despite this, no data is available on the effects of omalizumab in the treatment of EBP.

CONCLUSION

The current case is the first in our knowledge to be genetically confirmed as EBP and successfully treated with omalizumab. The diagnosis of EBP was initially challenging due to the late-onset presentation and lack of other supporting features such as nail dystrophy. The improvement in bullous skin lesions and disabling pruritus after omalizumab treatment further supports the etiopathological role of IgE. In patients with EBP, increased serum IgE in the absence of obvious allergic or parasitic disease may support the use of anti-IgE therapy when conventional therapy fails.

ACKNOWLEDGEMENT

The authors would like to acknowledge Dr Mansoor Ali Hameed for proofreading the manuscript. No funding organization or sponsoring body has been involved in the design and conduct of the study.

DISCLAIMER

This case report is published in J Clin Exp Dermatol Res. 2020;11:520. DOI: 10.35248/2155-9554.20.11.520 [*Citation:* Taha SA, Al-Nesf MA, Al-Obaidli AM (2020) Successful Treatment of Epidermolysis Bullosa Pruriginosa with Anti-IgE Therapy (Omalizumab): A Case Report and Four Years Follow Up. J Clin Exp Dermatol Res. 11:520. DOI: 10.35248/2155-9554.20.11.520]
Copyright: © 2020 Taha SA, et al. This is an open-access article distributed under the terms of the Creative Commons Attribution License, which permits unrestricted use, distribution, and reproduction in any medium, provided the original author and source are credited.

KEY MESSAGES

- Diagnosis of EBP can be challenging due to late-onset presentation and absence of other supporting features.
- Anti-IgE therapy may be useful in patients with EBP with increased serum IgE in the absence of obvious allergic or parasitic disease when conventional therapy fails.

REFERENCES

1. Shinkuma S. Dystrophic epidermolysis bullosa: a review. Clin Cosmet Investig Dermatol. 2015;8: 275-84.
2. Kim WB, Alavi A, Pope E, Walsh S. Epidermolysis bullosa pruriginosa: Case series and review of the literature. Int J Low Extrem Wounds. 2015;14:196-9.
3. Yang CS, Lu Y, Farhi A, Nelson Williams C, Kashgarian M, Glusac EJ, et al. An incompletely penetrant novel mutation in COL7A1 causes epidermolysis bullosa pruriginosa and dominant dystrophic epidermolysis bullosa phenotypes in an extended kindred. Pediatr Dermatol. 2012;29:725-31.
4. Vivehanantha S, Carr RA, McGrath JA, Taibjee SM, Madhogaria S, Ilchyshyn A. Epidermolysis bullosa pruriginosa: a case with prominent histopathologic inflammation. JAMA Dermatol. 2013;149: 727-31.
5. Maurer M, Altrichter S, Schmetzer O, Scheffel J, Church MK, Metz M. Immunoglobulin E-mediated autoimmunity. Front Immunol. 2018;9:689.

6. Dimson OG, Giudice GJ, Fu CI, Bergh FV, Warren SJ, Janson MM, et al. Identification of a potential effector function for IgE autoantibodies in the organ-specific autoimmune disease bullous pemphigoid. J Invest Dermatol. 2003;120:784-8.
7. Drera B, Castiglia D, Zoppi N, Gardella R, Tadni G, Floriddia G, et al. Dystrophic epidermolysis bullosa pruriginosa in Italy: clinical and molecular characterization. Clin Genet. 2006;70:339-47.
8. Tang MM, Leong KF, Cristina H. Dystrophic epidermolysis bullosa pruriginosa: the first report of a family in Malaysia. Med J Malaysia. 2013;68:81-5.
9. Brennan F. The pathophysiology of pruritus-A review for clinicians. Prog Palliat Care. 2016;24:133-46.
10. Koga H, Teye K, Yamashita K. Detection of anti-type VII collagen IgE antibodies in epidermolysis bullosa acquisita. Br J Dermatol. 2019;180:1107-13.
11. Kaplan AP, Giménez-Arnau AM, Saini SS. Mechanisms of action that contribute to efficacy of omalizumab in chronic spontaneous urticaria. Allergy. 2017;72:519-33.
12. Yalcin AD, Genc GE, Celik B, Gumuslu S. Anti-IgE monoclonal antibody (Omalizumab) is effective in treating bullous pemphigoid and its effects on soluble CD200. Clin Lab. 2014;60:523-4.

CASE 11

The Cause Behind Multiple Drug Hypersensitivity Reactions in a Patient with Atopic Dermatitis

Iman Nasr, Shamsa H Al Maawali, Prabha MP Liyanage

CASE PRESENTATION

A 39-year-old patient, with a background of DiGeorge syndrome (DGS) with hypocalcemia and epilepsy, was referred to the Immunology Department for evaluation of multiple allergies to oral calcium and multiple antiepileptics.

The patient had a long-standing history of atopic dermatitis with no trigger identified. According to his sister, he improves whenever he is off calcium supplements. As a result of stopping his calcium supplements, the patient had repeated admissions for hypocalcemia managed with intravenous calcium. Once this was switched to oral calcium, the patient reported generalized dermatitis after 2–3 days after which oral calcium was stopped. The impression was delayed allergic reaction to calcium and was kept on vitamin D with advice to increase his intake of dietary calcium with the help of the dietitian. Unfortunately, the patient developed seizures likely as a result of hypocalcemia. Electroencephalogram (EEG) revealed left-sided epileptic focal discharges for which he was started by the neurologist on oral carbamazepine. He was admitted 2 weeks later with severe generalized dermatitis and possibly impending Stevens–Johnson syndrome as per the dermatologist in view of burning sensation in the mouth but no mucosal lesions. He was afebrile and his laboratory parameters were normal. The drug was stopped immediately. After consultation with the neurologist, he was advised to change to topiramate; however, again after few days of treatment the patient presented with severe generalized erythema and the drug was stopped. This was then replaced by phenytoin with similar drug eruption. Finally, the patient was switched to levetiracetam 750 mg BID when he presented to the emergency department with features of DRESS (drug reaction with eosinophilia and systemic symptoms) syndrome. The patient was febrile. There was no mucosal involvement. Laboratory investigations revealed high eosinophils on full blood count and deranged liver function tests. Kidney function was normal. HIV and Hepatitis B and C screen was negative. The immunology team was consulted during this admission since it was recently established and there was no immunology service before.

On reviewing the patient's history of multiple allergies, the possibility of an excipient as a cause of these allergies was top on the list. A thorough search of all the ingredients in all the medications the patient received was done where the common ingredient in all the medications was a dye called sunset yellow (also known as FD&C 6 and E110). After recovery and as part of the workup, the patient had a patch test done in the hospital due to the high risk of developing DRESS to the calcium carbonate brand he was taking, levetiracetam, topiramate (10% dilution), calcitriol, and the dyes sunset yellow (FD&C 6, E110) and tartrazine (FD&C 5, E102) since both these dyes were present in the calcium carbonate brand. The result was read after 48 hours with erythema at the site of calcium carbonate and sunset yellow dye. It was negative to levetiracetam 500 mg (which was the only strength available at our pharmacy then) and topiramate. It was also negative to tartrazine and calcitriol. The conclusion was a delayed allergic reaction to sunset yellow. The patient was advised to avoid all products that contained this dye. He was switched to a calcium carbonate product that was free of sunset yellow with good tolerance. He was also carefully challenged with levetiracetam using the 250-mg dose which did not contain yellow sunset dye at graded doses using a slow delayed protocol until a full dose of 500 mg twice daily was reached with no reaction. The 500-mg dose also did not contain yellow sunset while the 750-mg dose did which explains his previous reaction when started on 750 mg. He was reviewed after 6 months and had no further episodes of atopic dermatitis. His calcium levels remained normal. His last EEG was reported as normal awake EEG for which the levetiracetam dose was further reduced to 250 mg twice daily which too did not contain sunset yellow.

DISCUSSION

DiGeorge syndrome or 22q11.2 deletion syndrome is one of the most common genetic microdeletion syndromes, which is usually diagnosed since early childhood.[1] It is associated with physical manifestations such as facial, velopharyngeal, cardiac, immunologic, and endocrinal abnormalities.[1,2] In addition, it is associated with neuropsychiatric manifestations such as intellectual disability, schizophrenia, depression, panic disorder, and attention-deficit/hyperactivity disorder.[1] Psychiatric manifestations are more obvious in undiagnosed patients at adulthood.[1] DGS is prone to seizures because of hypocalcemia, cortical agenesis, and rarely neural tube defects.[2] In dealing with any questionable allergy, it is found to be helpful to identify all the ingredients (active and nonactive) such as dyes in any suspected food or drug allergy.[3] The food-coloring history is related to early Egyptian and Roman civilizations, when they used natural coloring agents such as saffron, various flowers, carrots, mulberries, and beets.[4] Then, in the middle of the nineteenth century, new synthetic azo dye agents (–N=N–) were introduced and they were extensively used later on in canned and fast food.[4] They are indeed used to make food more attractive but have no nutritional or preservative value in them.[4]

Azo dyes are a family of dyes such as ponceau 4R (E124), indigo carmine (E132), azorubine (E122), tartrazine (E102), sunset yellow FCF (E110), Bordeaux red (E123), and sodium benzoate (E211).[5-7]

Sunset yellow (SY, E110, FD&C Yellow No. 6), as shown in **Figure 1**, is a disodium salt of 6-hydoxy-5-[(4-sulphophenyl)azo]-2-naphthalenesulfonic acid and it has a molecular weight of 452.36 g/mol.[4,8] It is orange yellow in color and has been used widely in food, cosmetic, and drug coloring.[4] In our patient, sunset yellow was found as an ingredient in calcium carbonate tablets, carbamazepine, phenytoin, topiramate, and levetiracetam 750 mg. Therefore, this dye was highly suspected as a cause for his reactions. His medications were replaced with brands and doses that did not contain sunset yellow. Levetiracetam 500 mg and 250 mg did

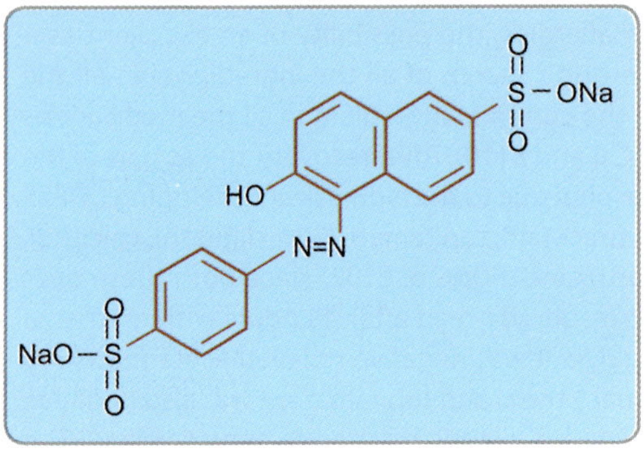

FIG. 1: Structure of sunset yellow dye.

not contain sunset yellow and therefore was tolerated well. This was also true with the new brand of calcium carbonate.

For each dye, there is an accepted daily intake (ADI) as per the international research and the recommendations of the Codex Committee on Food Additives and Contaminants (CCFAC). This daily dose should be strictly followed by the manufactures.[4,9] The ADI, which was established by the Joint FAO/WHO Expert Committee on Food Additives (1994) for sunset yellow, is 0–2.5 mg/kg body weight (bw)/day.[4,10] This was reduced to 0–1 mg/kg bw/day in 2009 in view of the adverse events related to sunset yellow.[10] However, after revisiting this safety concern, an evaluation was conducted by the Joint FAO/WHO Expert Committee on Food Additives and additional toxicological information made available where the European Food Safety Authority (EFSA) had established an ADI of 0–4 mg/kg bw/day for sunset yellow.

Sunset yellow is as common as tartrazine in causing allergy (in the form of urticaria, angioedema, allergic eosinophilic gastroenteritis, anaphylactic shock, vasculitis, and thromboxane synthesis inhibition), especially who is sensitive originally to paracetamol, acetylsalicylic acid, and sodium benzoate.[3,7] In addition, it uncommonly contributes to exacerbation of bronchoconstriction in asthmatic patients.[11] Even though, more studies are needed to evaluate the sunset yellow-related hypersensitivity reactions.

Many studies have proved that coloring agents are mutagenic and carcinogenic, as they are metabolized in the intestinal wall and liver to free aromatic amines.[4] Also, they cause suppression of the central nervous system (CNS).[4]

Sunset yellow dye was banned in some countries due to its mutagenicity while in others it is not, which may indicate that these agents have different effects on people depending on dose, age, gender, nutritional status, genetic factor, and time of exposure.[4] One plant bioassay study[4] has proved the genotoxic and cytotoxic impact of sunset yellow, especially with higher doses. This cytotoxicity and even carcinogenicity were supported by other studies.[7,12] Another study[13] has showed that sunset yellow changes the functional responses of splenocytes at noncytotoxic dose. Also, it has some adverse effects on several behavioral developmental parameters during the early lactation period.[8] In addition, it has been shown that these coloring agents damage and paint leukocytes of patients with bronchial asthma by trypan blue.[5] Indeed, antigen-specific damage of leukocytes may be used to determine the causative allergen.[5] It is also reported to reduce testes weight.[10] Hence, it is warranted to eliminate the undertested or low safety profile-coloring agents from the products.[7,12] Many methods were developed in order to determine these agents in the product and their levels as a preventive and monitoring measure.[6]

CONCLUSION

In patients with a history of multiple drug allergies, a detailed and thorough investigation into the ingredients of drugs, cosmetics, and food should be performed. While hypersensitivity reactions to dyes are uncommon, they still occur in a minority of people and can lead to consequences such as in our case uncontrolled hypocalcemia and epilepsy. The patient should be referred to a dietitian for guidance on avoidance of products containing the culprit dye.

KEY MESSAGES

- Always look into excipients in any case of multiple drug allergies.
- Allergy to additives and dyes is not uncommon and is worth exploring in all patients with atopic dermatitis, especially if severe or persistent.

REFERENCES

1. Kraus C, Vanicek T, Weidenauer A, Khanaqa T, Stamenkovic M, Lanzenberger R, et al. DiGeorge syndrome: Relevance of psychiatric symptoms in undiagnosed adult patients. Wien Klin Wochenschr. 2018;130:283-7.
2. Alkan G, Emiroglu MK, Kartal A. DiGeorge syndrome with sacral myelomeningocele and epilepsy. J Pediatr Neurosci. 2017;12:344-5.
3. Gross PA, Lance K, Whitlock RJ, Blume RS. Additive allergy: allergic gastroenteritis due to yellow dye #6. Ann Int Med. 1989;111:87-8.
4. Dwivedi K, Kumar G. Genetic damage induced by a food coloring dye (sunset yellow) on meristematic cells of Brassica campestris L. J Environ Public Health Volume. 2015;319727.
5. Titova N. 300 The method of antigen specific damage of leucocytes by food additives in patients with bronchial asthma. World Allergy Organ J. 2012;5(Suppl 2):S114.
6. Alp H, Baskan D, Yasar A, Yayli N, Ocak U, Ocak M. Simultaneous determination of sunset yellow FCF, allura red AC, quinoline yellow WS, and tartrazine in food samples by RP-HPLC. J Chem. 2018;6486250.
7. Gomes KMS, de Oliveira MVGA, de Sousa Carvalho FR, Menezes CC, Peron AP. Citotoxicity of food dyes sunset yellow (E-110), bordeaux red (E-123), and tatrazine yellow (E-102) on Allium cepa L. root meristematic cells. Food Sci Technol (Campinas). 2013;33(1). Available from http://dx.doi.org/10.1590/S0101-20612013005000012 [Last accessed October, 2020].
8. Wang M, Zhang J, Gao Y, Yang X, Gao Y, Zhao J. Determination of sunset yellow in soft drinks at attapulgite modified expanded graphite paste electrode. J Electrochem Soc. 2014;161:H86-91.
9. Ariffin Z, Badrun F, Salleh B. Investigation on the presence of sunset yellow and tartrazine in commercial beverages and quantitation using ion-pair formation and extraction. Schematic Scholar Corpus ID 99608164. [online] Available from https://pdfs.semanticscholar.org/b411/8882afbfd5e7389caf44df2dae98d6c96e05.pdf?_ga=2.90048338.858881538.1592309711-239104181.1539701213 [Last accessed October, 2020].
10. European Food Safety Authority (EFSA). Scientific opinion on the re-evaluation of Sunset Yellow ECF (E-110) as a food additive. EFSA J. 2009;7(11):1330.
11. Weber RW, Hoffman M, Raine Jr DA, Nelson HS. Incidence of bronchoconstriction due to aspirin, azo dyes, non-azo dyes, and preservatives in a population of perennial asthmatics. J Allergy Clin Immunol. 1979;64:32-7.
12. Kobylewski S, Jacobson MF. Toxicology of food dyes. Int J Occup Environ Health. 2012;18:220-46.
13. Yadav A, Kumar A, Tripathi A. Sunset yellow FCF, a permitted food dye, alters functional responses of splenocytes at non-cytotoxic dose. Toxicol Lett. 2012;217.

CASE 12

Severe Atopic Dermatitis: Fast Effectiveness and Safety of Dupilumab

Marisa Paulino, Célia Costa

CASE PRESENTATION

We present the case of a 34-year-old Caucasian female with the diagnosis of persistent moderate allergic rhinitis and atopic dermatitis since childhood. She had a slight improvement during puberty of atopic dermatitis symptoms, but after her first pregnancy (11 years ago), there was a severe worsening, and after the second pregnancy, she developed generalized severe Xerosis with extensive areas of lichenification, erythema, excoriations, crusting and, in a lesser extent, oozing. She also developed severe constant pruritus leading to sleep deprivation. These symptoms contributed to a poor quality of life with impairment in social and family relationships, decrease in self-esteem and, as she worked as secretary, absenteeism from work. During this time, she consulted several dermatologists and allergologists. Skin prick tests were positive to house dust mites and dog epithelium. Patch tests with Portuguese standard battery and cosmetic battery were negative. Immunomodulatory agents such as azathioprine and cyclosporine were tried for a period of 6 months each, but were ineffective in controlling the disease. She was treated with systemic corticosteroids daily (1 mg/kg/day) but was able to reduce to a maintenance dosage of prednisolone 5 mg/day. She tried several topical treatments including—pimecrolimus, mometasone, methylprednisolone, and betamethasone. High-dosage second-generation H1 antihistamines (4/day) were tried but failed to control pruritus. Six months prior to her first appointment in our outpatient clinic, she had frequent exacerbations, especially in the face area, leading her to increase corticosteroids dosage until 20 mg daily by her own initiative. There were side effects from prolonged corticotherapy such as increased appetite and weight.

At physical examination, she presented Cushingoid facies, generalized erythema, severe dry skin, crusting, and lichenification areas with predominance in the face—SCORing Atopic Dermatitis (SCORAD): 103.7, Eczema Area and Severity Index (EASI): 30, and Dermatology Life Quality Index (DLQI): 24. Significant laboratory findings were blood eosinophilia (700) and total immunoglobulin E (IgE) 5,000 IU/mL. A skin biopsy was performed compatible with atopic dermatitis.

She was proposed to start dupilumab and accepted after ophthalmology evaluation. At time of the first administration, she was medicated with—prednisolone 5 mg/day, topic pimecrolimus—10 mg/g, topic mometasone—1 mg/g on demand (daily, 2–3×/day), nasal fluticasone 27.5 µg 12/12h and emollients. Before the first administration of dupilumab, she presented SCORAD: 93, EASI: 33, and DLQI: 21. She started with a dosage of 600 mg, followed by 300 mg every 2 weeks. Systemic corticosteroids were suspended after the first administration. Significant clinical improvement at various levels was observed after two administrations and before the third administration of dupilumab; she had SCORAD: 43.5, EASI: 21.4, and DLQI: 4. After 16 weeks of treatment, she remained without corticotherapy, stopped the antihistamines, and reduced the usage of topic mometasone. She also reported absence of pruritus and a significant improvement in quality of sleep, with results of SCORAD: 42, EASI: 9.3, and DLQI: 6.

DISCUSSION

Atopic dermatitis (AD) is a debilitating chronic, relapsing disease characterized by intense pruritus and excoriations, with erythematous, Xerotic, lichenified, fissured skin, and increased risk of skin infections.[1,2] AD is often associated with sleep deprivation and social stigmatization that severely impacts the psychosocial wellbeing of both patients and their relatives.[3] AD is also associated with an increased economic burden derived from work and school absenteeism, reduced productivity, and health-related costs associated with medical visits and treatments.[3]

Most patients have their disease controlled with emollients, topical corticosteroids, topical immunomodulators, or phototherapy.[3,4] However, it is estimated that approximately 20% of patients have moderate-to-severe AD refractory to these treatments.[4] When systemic therapies are needed, choice was limited until now. Long-term use of corticosteroids is discouraged due to their side effects and rebound effects upon discontinuation.[4] Immunomodulators such as cyclosporine, azathioprine, methotrexate, and mycophenolate are commonly used; however, nearly half the patients must discontinue it due to ineffectiveness or side effects.[3]

Dupilumab is a humanized monoclonal antibody targeting—interleukin (IL)-4 and IL-13 receptors[1] that showed efficacy in patients with severe AD when other systemic therapies failed or were discontinued due to side effects. Clinical trials proved a significant improvement of symptoms and quality of life at 16 weeks of treatment (defined as a 75% reduction in EASI) and maintained until week 52.[1,5] Pruritus is reported to improve as early as 2 days. Dupilumab is generally well tolerated with trials showing similar incidence of adverse events as placebo.[1,5]

Our patient was suffering from side effects from previous therapies and dependent on corticotherapy unable to discontinue it. After starting dupilumab, she had a significant improvement of quality of life with a high reduction in EASI (72%), SCORAD (55%), and in DLQI of 71%, at week 16.

CONCLUSION

Patients with AD suffer from significant psychosocial effects that can lead to depression and anxiety-related disorders. This patient had severe constant pruritus that leads to sleep deprivation and skin lesions affecting the face that affected her work resulting in a lack of productivity and absenteeism. Dupilumab showed excellent result in controlling both skin lesions and pruritus, providing the patients with a better quality of life. Dupilumab was not only faster but more effective than previous therapies and allowed the discontinuation of corticosteroids.

KEY MESSAGES

- AD has a significant impact in mental and physical health.
- Pruritus is one of the most debilitating symptoms and often uncontrolled by antihistamines.
- Prolonged corticotherapy is not recommended due to side effects.
- Dupilumab proved a fast efficacy in patients with severe AD, since after the first administration, with a progressive improvement and safety during at least 52 weeks.

REFERENCES

1. Blauvelt A, de Bruin-Weller M, Gooderham M, Cather JC, Weisman J, Pariser D, et al. Long-term management of moderate-to-severe atopic dermatitis with dupilumab and concomitant topical corticosteroids (LIBERTY AD CHRONOS): A 1-year, randomised, double-blinded, placebo-controlled, phase 3 trial. Lancet. 2017;389(10086):2287-303.
2. Ferrucci S, Casazza G, Angileri L, Tavecchio S, Germiniasi F, Berti E, et al. Clinical Response and Quality of Life in Patients with Severe Atopic Dermatitis Treated with Dupilumab: A Single-Center Real Life Experience. J Clin Med. 2020;9(3):791.
3. Ariens LFM, Bakker DS, van der Schaft J, Garritsen FM, Thijs JL, de Bruin-Weller MS. Dupilumab in atopic dermatitis: rationale, latest evidence and place in therapy. Ther Adv Chronic Dis. 2018;9(9):159-70.
4. Wu J, Guttman-Yassky E. Efficacy of biologics in atopic dermatitis. Expert Opin Biol Ther. 2020;20(5):525-38.
5. Wang FP, Tang XJ, Wei CQ, Xu LR, Mao H, Luo FM, et al. Dupilumab treatment in moderate-to-severe atopic dermatitis: A systematic review and meta-analysis. J Dermatol Sci. 2018;90(2):190-8.

CASE 13

Role of Patch Testing in Atopic Dermatitis

Michael Rudenko

CASE PRESENTATION

A 40-year-old male patient presented to our department with a history of dermatitis that started to get worse in December; it affected mainly his torso and neck. He developed an infection and had treatment with oral antibiotics as well as steroid creams.

We have arranged patch testing that showed positive results to Nickel sulfate, Potassium dichromate, formaldehyde, imidazolidinyl urea (Germall 115), 2-bromo-2-nitropropane-1,3-diol (bronopol), and irritation with gold sodium thiosulfate.

We also advised to use Reveal and Conceal to check all metal objects in the house. Continued with very good skincare as well as restricted use of steroid creams under the supervision of dermatologist.

The test showed positive for nickel on his metal showerhead. He has since started to use another shower and his symptoms have resolved. We have subsequently clarified his history and the aggravation of his symptoms happened at the time the new shower was installed.

DISCUSSION

Differentiating the two diseases, allergic contact dermatitis and atopic dermatitis, is important for successful treatment. Both conditions have a significant negative impact on quality of life (QOL) and are a significant clinical problem in both children and adults.[1]

The pathogenesis of atopic dermatitis is multifactorial and complex. It involves defects related to epidermal barrier and immunological dysfunction. Some patients have filaggrin gene null mutations inherited by an autosomal semidominant fashion. Penetration of allergens is increased in patients with atopic dermatitis. These pathological changes with frequent use of emollients and topical medications may increase the risk of allergic contact dermatitis.[2]

Allergic contact dermatitis is a classic type IV hypersensitivity reaction, caused by a delayed-type hypersensitivity response to contact allergens driven by activation of naïve T cells, leading to differentiation of memory T cells specific to the chemicals. Contact allergy is an important comorbidity and has potential to exacerbate atopic dermatitis.[2]

CONCLUSION

This case confirms the importance of patch testing to exclude contact allergy in patients with dermatitis. It is advisable to use patch testing when local treatment does not lead to improvement, or prior to systemic immunosuppressive treatment and use of biologics.

> **KEY MESSAGES**
> - Patch testing is useful for excluding contact allergy in patients with dermatitis.
> - Patch testing can be used when local treatment does not result in improvement, or before initiation of treatment with systemic immunosuppressive agents and biologics.

REFERENCES

1. Beattie PE, Lewis-Jones MS. A comparative study of impairment of quality of life in children with skin disease and children with other chronic childhood diseases. Br J Dermatol. 2006;155(1):145-51.

2. Owen JL, Vakharia PP, Silverberg JI. The role and diagnosis of allergic contact dermatitis in patients with atopic dermatitis. Am J Clin Dermatol. 2018;19(3):293-302.

CASE 14

Eczema Herpeticum in a Patient with Atopic Dermatitis during Treatment with Selective JAK1 Inhibitor: A Case Report

Michał Adamczyk, Bartłomiej Wawrzycki, Joanna Bartosińska, Dorota Krasowska

CASE PRESENTATION

A 19-year old male patient with a history of atopic dermatitis (AD) since infancy was admitted to Department of Dermatology, Venereology, and Pediatric Dermatology on August 2019, due to sudden appearance of multiple, small, umbilicated, painful vesicles, and erosions disseminated within whole body surface area (**Figs. 1A** to **D**). Among concomitant diseases, he also reported atopic asthma and Gilbert syndrome, but he was never diagnosed with eczema herpeticum (EH) and reported no symptoms caused by herpes simplex viruses before. On clinical examination, painful, symmetric lymphadenopathy in axillar and inguinal regions was also present but he was otherwise in good condition and did not complain of any general symptoms.

Due to the severe course of AD in the past, the subject was treated with cyclosporine A for >1 year (2015–2016) with good tolerance, but only partial improvement of AD skin lesions. In December 2018, he was qualified for clinical trial evaluating the safety and efficacy of selective Janus kinase (JAK1) inhibitor. After a 12-week blinded treatment period, during which he may have been given study drug or placebo, he received a full dose of the investigational drug. He then continued therapy for the next 6 months with good tolerance and excellent improvement of AD skin lesions until he was admitted for current hospitalization.

The diagnosis of EH was established based on clinical findings. Laboratory tests revealed slightly elevated C-reactive protein and total bilirubin levels (6.9 mg/L and 2.36 mg/dL, respectively); complete blood count was within normal limits. Investigational drug was permanently discontinued, and the patient was treated with high doses of intravenous aciclovir (10 mg/kg/day for 10 days) and topical antiseptics with gradual improvement. The subject was discharged from hospital, and 3 weeks later, he experienced another episode of EH with more limited lesions involving the trunk for which he was not hospitalized and was successfully controlled with oral aciclovir 400 mg five times per day administered for 10 days.

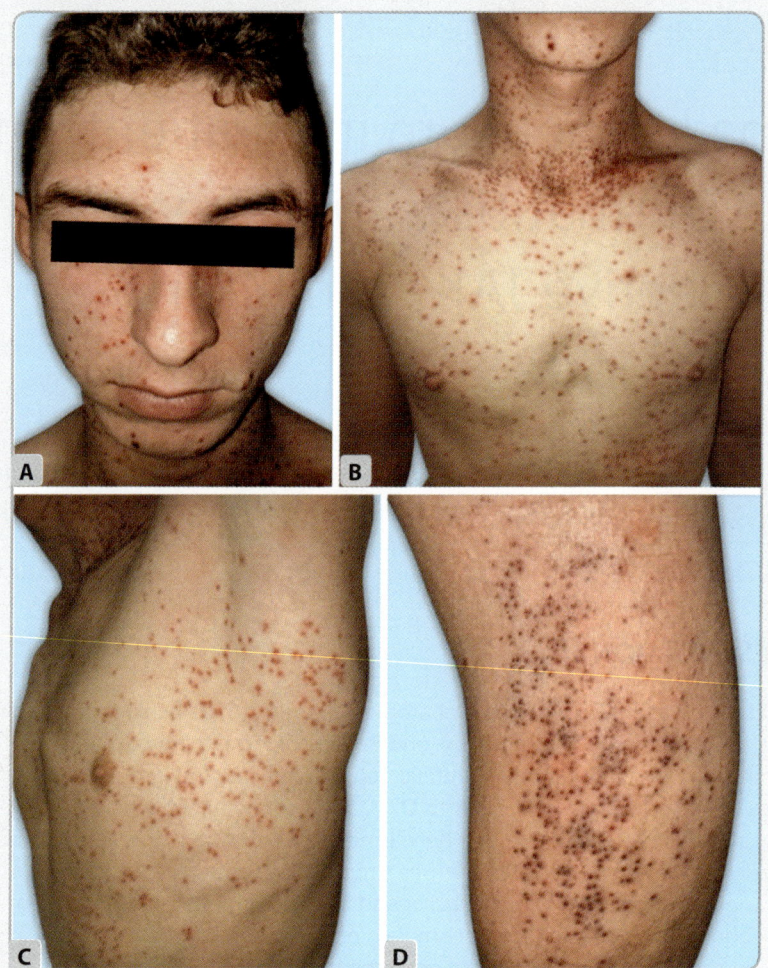

FIGS. 1A TO D: Skin lesions of eczema herpeticum on the day of admission to hospital.

DISCUSSION

Eczema herpeticum (EH) is a potentially life-threatening infection caused by herpes simplex viruses (HSV) 1 and 2. It was first described by Kaposi[1] in 1887, which is the reason for the alternative name of the entity—"Kaposi varicelliform eruption," commonly used in literature. AD is the most frequent underlying skin condition in patients with EH; however, many other dermatoses may predispose to it, including but not limited to—Darier-White disease, pemphigus foliaceus, mycosis fungoides, Sézary syndrome, ichthyosis vulgaris, Hailey–Hailey disease, and burns.[2] According to some authors, the term EH should be restricted to patients with the concomitant eczematous disease, whereas Kaposi varicelliform eruption to all other patients with typical clinical manifestations.[3] Because of its rarity, no epidemiological data concerning frequency of the entity are available; however, according to some estimations, it may affect 3% of patients with AD during their lifetime.[4]

Clinical manifestation of EH includes multiple, small, and umbilicated vesicles;[5]

after several days, vesicles evolve into erosions covered by crusts. Most frequent locations include head, neck, and upper trunk. However, any location may be affected. Skin symptoms are usually accompanied by fever, malaise, and lymphadenopathy.[6] Viremia with multiple organ involvement and encephalitis may occur, especially in immunocompromised individuals, and mortality rates range from 10 to 50%[3] and were as high as 80% before the era of antiviral drugs.[2]

The pathogenesis of EH is still not fully understood. Both HSV1 and HSV2 may be responsible for the appearance of skin lesions, and a higher incidence of HSV1 is associated with a greater prevalence of this subtype in the general population. EH may occur as a result of primary or secondary HSV infection.[5]

The diagnosis of EH is mainly clinical; however, some additional laboratory tests may be needed to confirm the diagnosis [e.g., Tzanck smear, direct fluorescent antibody staining, viral antigen detection, and polymerase chain reaction (PCR)]. Complete blood count, erythrocyte sedimentation rate (ESR), and C-reactive protein may reveal features of systemic infection. Skin swabs may confirm superinfection with *Staphylococcus aureus* or other bacteria. Differential diagnoses include widespread impetigo, eczema vaccinatum, chickenpox, and contact dermatitis.[2] When ocular or neurological involvement is suspected, patient should be consulted by an appropriate specialist to exclude viral keratitis and encephalitis.[7]

The most important in clinical management is to use antiviral agents as early as possible to avoid systemic complications. Aciclovir is a systemic agent of choice in the treatment of EH. As a nucleoside analog, it interferes with viral DNA synthesis only in HSV-infected cells in a monophosphate form. It is very effective and safe; the ability of aciclovir to shorten the duration of EH was proved in a randomized, double-blind, placebo-controlled clinical trial.[8] Recommended doses are 5–10 mg/kg three times per day in intravenous infusions administered for 7 days or longer, depending on clinical evaluation. In mild cases, oral administration is sufficient.[2] In cases of recurrent EH, long-term prophylaxis should be considered with oral doses of aciclovir of 400 mg twice daily.[7] Other systemic antiviral therapies, which may be recommended, include valacyclovir, famciclovir, penciclovir, and foscarnet.[2]

In the case of bacterial superinfection, systemic and topical antibiotics may be needed and sometimes they are used routinely as prophylaxis. The topical use of antiseptic lotions may be beneficial by drying out vesicles and preventing superinfection.[2] Due to lack of evidence about the effectiveness and potential risk of provoking contact allergy, topical forms of aciclovir and other antivirals are not recommended in the treatment of EH, except cases with ocular and mucosal involvement.

Many predisposing factors for EH were found in AD population. Impaired skin barrier makes penetration of HSV to the skin easier. Nectin 1, a desmosomal protein, was identified as an important receptor for the viruses in the skin. Additionally, the predominance of Th2 response, typically observed in AD patients, lowers innate response against HSV. Another important predisposing factor includes deficiency of cathelicidin (LL-37), an antimicrobial peptide in the epidermis. Finally, impaired production of type 1 interferons α and β, mainly due to deficiency of plasmacytoid dendritic cells, was observed in AD skin, and this type of interferons exhibits strong antiviral properties.[2] Polymorphisms of many different genes, including filaggrin, interferons, and thymic stromal lymphopoietin (TSLP), were found to be associated with higher risk of developing EH in AD patients.[4]

Regarding the influence of current therapy on the risk of EH, literature data present equivocal results. Among topical treatments, only calcineurin inhibitors, tacrolimus and pimecrolimus, are suspected to increase susceptibility to viral complications. No data exist about negative impact of corticosteroids.[4] Interestingly, treatment with systemic cyclosporine A, another calcineurin inhibitor with strong immunosuppressive properties, was not found to increase the risk of infectious complications in subjects with AD, including EH.[9] Moreover, a recent meta-analysis of randomized control studies did not prove the association between dupilumab, a first biologic drug inhibiting interleukins 4 and 13, and the risk of infections.[10]

JAK inhibitors include many different small-molecule drugs, among which nine are being currently investigated in the treatment of AD as both systemic and topical therapies. Inhibition of tyrosine kinases results with blocking signal transmission and activation of immune cells. They differ from the exact spectrum of inhibited JAK kinases (**Table 1**). They showed excellent efficacy in the treatment of many different conditions, including hematologic malignancies, autoimmune diseases, and AD.[11] Several of JAK inhibitors, including systemic upadacitinib, abrocitinib, and topical ruxolitinib, are on late stages of development in AD and are expected to be approved in the near future. The first two, due to excellent efficacy and safety profile, were granted breakthrough therapy for AD by FDA.[12] In other diseases, including rheumatoid arthritis, psoriatic arthritis, and ulcerative colitis, treatment with JAK inhibitors was found to be associated with higher (comparable with biologics) risk of serious infections, especially reactivation of varicella–herpes zoster virus (VZV).[13] To date, no elevated risk of serious infections was detected during treatment of AD with this group of drugs.

In our case, the subject did not report HSV lesions in the past. An episode of EH was probably a feature of primary infection. We cannot exclude the possible influence of concomitant therapy with JAK inhibitor. Fortunately, the drug was immediately discontinued, and proper therapy was given with good outcome.

CONCLUSION

Modern therapies with small-molecule JAK inhibitors are highly effective in the treatment of AD. However, we should not forget about immunosuppression associated with therapy, thus, particular caution should be given during treatment.

TABLE 1: Janus kinase (JAK) inhibitors currently investigated in atopic dermatitis.

Drug name	Mode of action	Phase of studies	Drug form
Upadacitinib	Selective anti-JAK1	III	Oral
Abrocitinib	Selective anti-JAK1	III	Oral
Baricitinib	Anti-JAK1 and JAK2	III	Oral
Gusacitinib	Anti-JAK1-3, anti-SYK	II	Oral
Ruxolitinib	Anti-JAK1 and JAK2	III	Topical
Delgocitinib	Anti JAK1-3, anti-TYK	II	Topical
Brepocitinib	Anti-JAK1, anti-TYK	II	Topical
ATI-502	Anti-JAK1 and JAK3	II	Topical
Tofacitinib	Anti-JAK1 and JAK3	II	Topical

(SYK: spleen tyrosine kinase; TYK: tyrosine kinase)

KEY MESSAGE

- Systemic immunosuppressive therapies, including JAK inhibitors, may carry a risk of infectious complications in subjects with AD.

REFERENCES

1. Kaposi M. Pathologie und Therapie der Hautkrankheiten. Vienna, Urban and Schwarzenberg; 1887.
2. Wollenberg A. Eczema herpeticum. Chem Immunol Allergy. 2012;96:89-95.
3. Wollenberg A, Wetzel S, Burgdorf WH, Haas J. Viral infections in atopic dermatitis: pathogenic aspects and clinical management. J Allergy Clin Immunol. 2003;112(4):667-74.
4. Damour A, Garcia M, Seneschal J, Lévêque N, Bodet C. Eczema Herpeticum: Clinical and Pathophysiological Aspects. Clin Rev Allergy Immunol. 2020;59(1):1-18.
5. Wollenberg A, Zoch C, Wetzel S, Plewig G, Przybilla B. Predisposing factors and clinical features of eczema herpeticum: a retrospective analysis of 100 cases. J Am Acad Dermatol. 2003;49(2):198-205.
6. Wheeler CE Jr, Abele DC. Eczema herpeticum, primary and recurrent. Arch Dermatol. 1966;93(2):162-73.
7. Rerinck HC, Kamann S, Wollenberg A. Eczema herpeticatum: Pathogenese und Therapie. Hautarzt. 2006;57(7):586-91.
8. Niimura M, Nishikawa T, Martin A, Booth A, Brocklehurst P, Kinghorn G, et al. Treatment of eczema herpeticum with oral acyclovir. Am J Med. 1988;85(2A):49-52.
9. Kim SW, Park YW, Kwon IH, Kim KH. Cyclosporin treatment of atopic dermatitis: is it really associated with infectious diseases? Ann Dermatol. 2010;22(2):170-2.
10. Fleming P, Drucker AM. Risk of infection in patients with atopic dermatitis treated with Dupilumab: a meta-analysis of randomized controlled trials. J Am Acad Dermatol. 2018;78(1):62-9.e61.
11. Arora CJ, Khattak FA, Tahir YM, Bukola Mary I, Stephen S. The effectiveness of JAK inhibitors in treating atopic dermatitis: a systematic review and meta-analysis. Dermatol Ther. 2020;e13685.
12. Rodrigues MA, Torres T. JAK/STAT inhibitors for the treatment of atopic dermatitis. J Dermatolog Treat. 2020;31(1):33-40.
13. Alten R, Mischkewitz M, Stefanski AL, Dörner T. Janus kinase inhibitors: State of the art in clinical use and future perspectives. Z Rheumatol. 2020;79(3):241-54.

CASE 15

Dupilumab-induced Face Dermatitis in Patients with Adult-onset Atopic Dermatitis and Severe Asthma

Mona Al-Ahmad, Eman Alsayed, Wafaa Talaat

CASE PRESENTATION

A 25-year old female presented to allergy clinic with adult-onset atopic dermatitis and severe asthma. She had childhood-onset asthma, which was diagnosed earlier as severe allergic asthma, with recurrent exacerbations that required maximal medical therapy, including high-dose inhaled corticosteroids plus long-acting B2 agonist [Global Initiative for Asthma (GINA) guidelines)].[1] Her asthma remained uncontrolled and required multiple short courses of oral corticosteroids (OCS) for excarnations.

Her atopic dermatitis,[2] on the other hand, was diagnosed 2 years ago with widespread skin lesions throughout her body. She received several courses of topical corticosteroids and topical calcineurin inhibitors, as well as systemic corticosteroids. She refused immunosuppressant therapy. She had no past medical history and was not on any systemic drugs. Her skin symptoms included intense itching, burning, and erythematous eczema at flexural areas of arms, legs, and trunk area, but spared the head and neck. On physical examination, she had severe eczematous lesions, lichenification, and follicular accentuation of arms, wrist, legs, back, and buttock area. Her average score on SCORing Atopic Dermatitis (SCORAD) was 71. The rest of her physical examination showed a respiratory rate of 20 and scattered wheezes bilaterally. Her investigations showed a normal complete blood count (CBC), white blood cell (WBC) count, normal C-reactive protein (CRP), total immunoglobulin E (IgE) of 1,200 kU/L, and skin prick test was positive to common outdoor aeroallergens (Bermuda and Salsola).

She was started on dupilumab[3] for both her adult-onset severe atopic dermatitis and severe asthma on April 2019. Initially, she had impressive improvement in all her atopic dermatitis lesions and her asthma control, but then she developed face dermatitis and erythema after about 12 weeks of dupilumab treatment. Concomitant treatment included topical corticosteroids and topical calcineurin inhibitors, but no systemic immunosuppressants. Her skin involvement showed sharply demarcated, itchy erythematous lesions in the head and neck area with no scaling, and this was different from her regular eczema. Treatment of erythema with topical and systemic drugs, including potent topical corticosteroids, topical calcineurin inhibitors, emollients, antifungal medication, antibiotics, antihistamines and oral corticosteroids, was unsuccessful. Although her lesions were persistent and did not respond to dupilumab treatment, she continued her dupilumab treatment. However, she experienced a general improvement in her eczema with improved skin lesions, itch and erythema, as well as her asthma severity, with less asthma exacerbations and better symptom control. Her SCORAD improved from 71 to 45.

DISCUSSION

Dupilumab is the first biologic registered for treatment of moderate-to-severe atopic dermatitis.[3] By binding to the interleukin (IL)-4 receptor alpha chain, dupilumab blocks IL-4 and IL-13 signaling, thereby modulating the T-helper (Th)2-mediated inflammation in atopic dermatitis. In clinical trials, conjunctivitis, herpes infections, and injection–site reactions were found to be the most frequently observed side effects.[3]

We describe a case of dupilumab-induced erythema and dermatitis in the head and neck distribution that developed in a patient with adult onset atopic dermatitis and severe asthma. She developed this erythema in a head and neck distribution, which was different from her usual atopic dermatitis lesions. The clinical manifestation included a sharply demarcated,[4] itchy erythema on the face and neck region, but not other sites of body. However, she had an overall good response to dupilumab, both in terms of her improved atopic dermatitis lesions and her severe asthma.

Adult-onset atopic dermatitis appears to be associated with a different disease phenotype[2] compared with childhood-onset atopic dermatitis. A differential diagnosis must be considered[5] in a patient presenting with an adult-onset eczematous eruption, including allergic contact dermatitis, mycosis fungoides/cutaneous T-cell lymphoma, psoriasis, scabies, drug-induced photosensitivity reaction, and others. A patch test with different panels of cosmetics and others was negative; a sunscreen patch test was negative as well. She had no history of using any photosensitive drugs and influence of ultraviolet radiation on the erythema was denied. There are some reported cases of similar observations during dupilumab use.[4]

CONCLUSION

This case describes dupilumab-induced face dermatitis in a patient with adult-onset atopic dermatitis and severe asthma, indicating the need to look for such induced reaction in patients receiving dupilumab treatment.

KEY MESSAGES

- Dupilumab is a dual cytokine inhibitor of IL-4 and IL-13 that has been recently approved for patients with moderate–severe atopic dermatitis.
- Physicians should be aware of potential effect of dupilumab-induced face dermatitis in patients with atopic dermatitis.

REFERENCES

1. http://ginaasthma.org
2. Toppila-Salmi S, Chanoine S, Karjalainen J, Pekkanen J, Bousquet J, Siroux V. Risk of adult-onset asthma increases with the number of allergic multimorbidities and decreases with age. Allergy. 2019;74(12):2406-16.
3. Beck LA, Thaci D, Hamilton JD, Graham NM, Bieber T, Rocklin R, et al. Dupilumab treatment in adults with moderate-to-severe atopic dermatitis. N Engl J Med. 2014;371:130-9.
4. de Wijs LEM, Nguyen NT, Kunkeler ACM, Nijsten T, Damman J, Hijnen DJ, et al. Clinical and histopathological characterization of paradoxical head and neck erythema in patients with atopic dermatitis treated with dupilumab: A case series. Br J Dermatol. 2020;183(4):745-9.
5. So JK, Hamstra A, Calame A, Hamann CR. Another great imitator: allergic contact dermatitis differential diagnosis, clues to diagnosis, histopathology, and treatment. Curr Treat Opt Allergy. 2015;2:333-48.

CASE 16

Dupilumab in the Treatment of Severe Atopic Dermatitis and Eczema Herpeticum Refractory to Systemic Treatment

Omar Lupi, Solange Oliveira Rodrigues Valle

CASE PRESENTATION

A 28-year-old man was admitted to our outpatient clinic (the Section of Immunology) for evaluation of photophobia and a painful vesicular and pustular rash on his right periocular area with eyelid involvement. The clinical examination showed vesicular, pustular, and crusty lesions on the right periocular area and eyelids (**Fig. 1**). The patient has had (A) atopic dermatitis (AD) diagnosis since the childhood and was previously treated with systemic corticosteroids, methotrexate, azathioprine, and cyclosporine in different regimens during his life. The skin examination showed

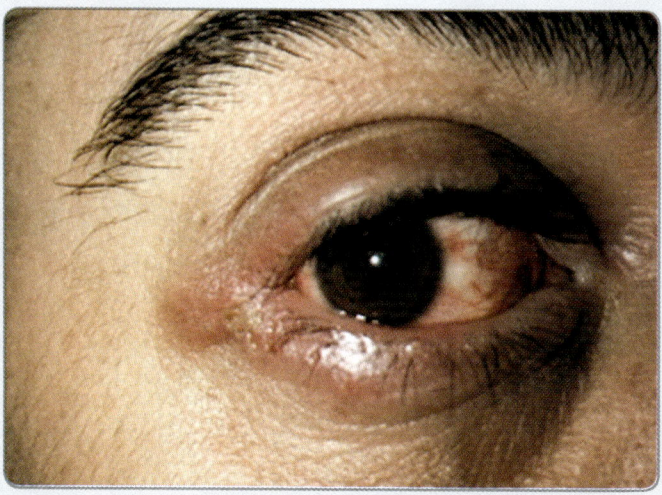

FIG. 1: Recurrent herpetic blepharoconjunctivitis in an atopic dermatitis patient.

extensive eczema affecting 90% of the skin tissue, along with very intense pruritus and dry skin, and a SCORing Atopic Dermatitis (SCORAD) of 88. There were widespread erythematosquamous plaques over the face, neck, and on the flexural surface of the upper and lower extremities.

Laboratory studies showed an erythrocyte sedimentation rate of 25 mm/h. The other hematologic values, serum enzyme levels, liver function tests, total protein, blood proteinogram (alpha-1-, alpha-2-, beta-, and gamma-globulins), urea, creatinine, and blood sugar levels were all normal. His immunoglobulin E (IgE) serum level was high at 1,200 kU/L (normal values <100 kU/L). An ophthalmologic examination revealed herpetic conjunctivitis and keratitis of the right eye. The neurological status was normal.

Treatment with oral valacyclovir 500 mg (two times) twice a day over a 7-week period did not improved the patient's condition. Ocular therapy with aciclovir ointment 5% applied five times a day for 7 days was also prescribed with only a partial response. The ophthalmologic examination after 2 weeks of the systemic and local treatment showed active herpetic infection but no dendritic scars were identified in the cornea. Follow-up examinations were carried out in the 1st, 2nd, and 3rd months after initial symptoms with no response to antiviral therapy. The disease remained poorly controlled, and the patient had very poor quality of life.

After the dupilumab results were published and the monoclonal antibody was approved in different countries, including Brazil, it was indicated for this patient. In March 2019, the patient received her first dose of 600 mg dupilumab, subcutaneously. The loading dose was followed by 300 mg every other week. Methotrexate was discontinued 2 months after dupilumab was introduced. In the fifth dose, the patient was already showing considerable improvement of AD lesions and EH was completely under control (**Fig. 2**). The current SCORAD is 8 after 1 year of dupixent therapy (**Fig. 3**). Desloratadine, topical corticosteroid, and the antidepressants have been discontinued, as well as all antiherpetic regimens.

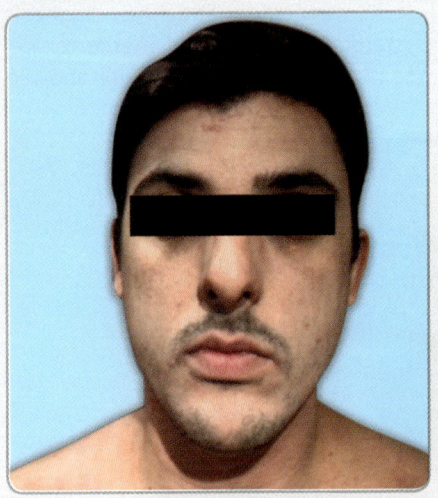

FIG. 2: Atopic dermatitis after 2 months of dupilumab treatment.

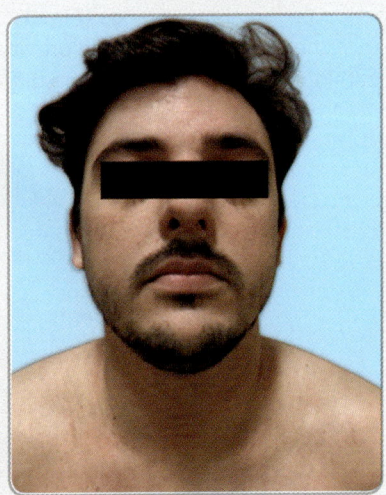

FIG. 3: 1-year follow-up of an atopic dermatitis patient after dupilumab (SCORAD: 8).

DISCUSSION

Eczema herpeticum (EH) is commonly associated to atopic dermatitis.[1] In milder cases, the skin symptoms are often restricted to the face with eye involvement and herpes simplex viruses (HSV) 1 is the main cause of EH. It is a dermatological emergency causing a mortality of up to 10% if untreated.[2] It frequently presents in a localized form and rarely disseminates via hematogenous spread with pulmonary, hepatic, ocular, and neurological manifestations.[1,2] Although it commonly appears on a background of atopic dermatitis (AD), many other dermatological conditions such as Darier's disease, thermal burns, pemphigus vulgaris, ichthyosis, mycosis fungoides, and Wiskott–Aldrich syndrome have been described preceding EH.[2] However, ADs are particularly susceptible to HSV infections and may develop disseminated EH. These patients usually have severe and bilateral herpetic ocular disease. Recent findings suggest that an increased number of IL-4 secreting cells can be cloned from lesions of AD.[3] IL-4 is a known Th1 cell inhibitor, and so theoretically, it could downregulate the immune response to HSV by inhibiting the Th1 cells.[3] Impairment of cell-mediated immunity in AD was suggested by the limited response to concanavalin A.[4] The reduced numbers of circulating natural killer cells and a decrease in IL-2 receptors during early EH contribute to the susceptibility of children with AD to cutaneous HSV infections. Here, we report a case of EH with unilateral ocular involvement.[3,4]

The question of ocular involvement in patients with EH and treated with dupilumab is very interesting, because 50% of patients with herpetic blepharoconjunctivitis (HB) may have corneal infections. The most common corneal lesions are vascular proliferation, necrosis, scaring, and ulceration.[1] Dupilumab has reported possible ocular side effects such as conjunctivitis, blepharitis, keratitis, eye pruritus and dry eye.[3,4] Herpes virus infection appears to be slightly increased overall in AD patients on dupilumab.[3] The decision to start dupilumab in our patient was not easy but the response was very effective for both AD and EH with HB. Dupilumab may have a protective effect against the incidence of EH but the mechanism is still unclear. Th2 immunity may not contribute significantly to the antiviral response, but other IL-4-producing cell such as natural killer T cells do have antiviral activity.

CONCLUSION

This is a case of localized EH in a severe AD patient, with unilateral ocular involvement and no response to combined systemic and topical antiherpetic therapy. Complete control of EH and a marked decrease of AD SCORAD was achieved after dupilumab therapy was started.

KEY MESSAGES

- Recurrent EH is commonly observed in severe AD patients.
- Herpetic blepharoconjunctivitis is a common complication of EH.
- Dupilumab is often associated with conjunctivitis.
- Despite of this, we describe a case of recurrent EH that was controlled after dupilumab.

REFERENCES

1. Darji K, Frisch S, Adjei Boakye E, Siegfried E. Characterization of children with recurrent eczema herpeticum and response to treatment with interferon-gamma. Pediatr Dermatol. 2017;34(6):686-9.
2. Amastu A, Yoshida M. Detection of Herpes simplex virus DNA in non-herpetic areas of patients with eczema herpeticum. Dermatol. 2000;200(2):104-7.
3. Akinlade B, Guttman-Yassky E, de Bruin-Weller M, Simpson EL, Blauvelt A, Cork MJ, et al. Conjunctivitis in dupilumab clinical trials. Br J Dermatol. 2019;181(3):459-73.
4. Treister AD, Kraff-Cooper C, Lio PA. Risk Factors for Dupilumab-associated Conjunctivitis in Patients with Atopic Dermatitis. JAMA Dermatol. 2018;154(10):1208-11.

CASE 17

Red Face during Dupilumab Therapy

E Serra-Baldrich, V Flores–Climent, J Spertino, L Puig

CASE PRESENTATION

A woman in her 40s was referred to the dermatology department for erythema affecting the head and neck region.

Her medical history was remarkable for asthma, rhinitis, and uncontrollable atopic dermatitis (AD) since she was 3 years old.

Her past treatments included antihistamines, topical and oral corticosteroids, topical immunomodulators, and oral immunosuppressants such as cyclosporine, azathioprine, and mofetil mycophenolate. The patient also underwent treatment with narrowband UVB phototherapy.

No sustained response was achieved with none of these treatments, so subcutaneous dupilumab (300 mg every 2 weeks) was started.

Dermatitis and pruritus greatly improved [decrease in Eczema Area and Severity Index (EASI), SCORing Atopic Dermatitis (SCORAD), and Dermatology Life Quality Index (DLQI) scales] 6 weeks after the first dose of dupilumab. During the follow-up, the patient presented cutaneous pruritic and burning lesions in her face.

Physical examination revealed patchy scaling erythema affecting the face and neck regions, no others lesions were observed (**Fig. 1**).

She related it to dupilumab and appeared 8 weeks after the first injection. The patch test was performed ruling out any superimposed allergic contact dermatitis. Treatment with topical pimecrolimus with narrowband ultraviolet B (UVB) was started with partial improvement of the lesions.

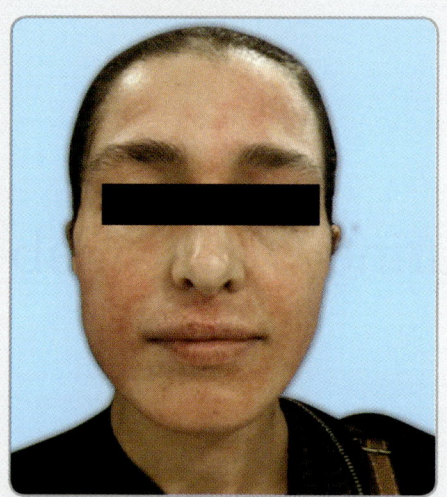

FIG. 1: Patchy scaling erythema on face and neck.

DISCUSSION

We report a patient presenting with a paradoxical head erythema, which appeared 8 weeks after start of dupilumab treatment.

The patient presented a demarcated, patchy erythema in her face area that showed scaling and experienced symptoms of itch and burning, although this was different from her pre-existent facial atopic dermatitis (AD).

The patient did not want to discontinue dupilumab treatment because of great improvement to the rest of her body. Unsuccessful treatments to date include topical corticosteroids, topical calcineurin inhibitors, moisturizers, oral prednisone, oral immunosuppressant, fluconazole, and ultraviolet B (UVB).

Dupilumab is the first biologic registered for treatment of moderate-to-severe AD. A fully human monoclonal antibody that binds to the IL-4 receptor alpha chain, blocking IL-4, and IL-13 signaling, thereby modulating the T-helper type 2-mediated inflammation in AD.[1]

Commonly reported adverse effects include conjunctivitis, herpes infections, headache, nasopharyngitis, and injection site reactions. More rare adverse effects described are alopecia areata, and ectropion.

There are few cases reported about this reaction.[2,3] Blocking the Th2 pathway could hypothetically result in a shift toward a more Th1-/Th17-/Th22-dominated response, resulting in the psoriasiform reaction pattern that Fowler et al. recently reported[4] during dupilumab treatment in two patients, but these were not located in the head and neck region. In other case report, facial redness is considered to be caused by hypersensitivity to *Malassezia* species and treatment with itraconazole could be recommended.[5]

Because this paradoxical erythema was only in a typical head and neck distribution, the possibility of an allergic contact dermatitis, *Malassezia furfur*-associated dermatitis, or a *Demodex*-associated rosacea-like dermatitis was also considered. Patch testing for allergic contact dermatitis was performed in our patient during dupilumab treatment with negative results.

We considered that this paradoxical head and neck erythema is a dupilumab-induced skin reaction and we think that further research is needed to elucidate this underlying pathophysiological process.

KEY MESSAGES

- Dupilumab is effective for the treatment of moderate-to-severe AD.
- Paradoxical erythema with dupilumab needs further research for understanding the pathophysiological process.

REFERENCES

1. Albader SS, Alharbi AA, Alenezi RF, Alsaif FM. Dupilumab side effect in a patient with atopic dermatitis: a case report study. Biologics. 2019;13:79-82.
2. Dalia Y, Marchese Johnson S. First reported case of facial rash after dupilumab therapy. Pract Dermatol. 2018;15:25-6.
3. de Wijs LEM, Nguyen NT, Kunkeler ACM, Nijsten T, Damman J, Hijnen DJ. Clinical and histopathological characterization of paradoxical head and neck erythema in atopic dermatitis patients treated with dupilumab: a case series. Br J Dermatol. 2020;183(4): 745-9.
4. Fowler E, Silverberg JI, Fox JD, Yosipovitch G. Presentation of Psoriasiform Dermatitis After Initiation of Treatment With Dupilumab for Atopic Dermatitis. Dermatitis. 2019;30(3):234-6.
5. de Beer FSA, Bakker DS, Haeck I, Ariens L, van der Schaft J, van Dijk MR, et al. Dupilumab facial redness: Positive effect of itraconazole. JAAD Case Rep. 2019;5(10):888-91.

CASE 18

A Case Report of a Patient with Refractory Severe Atopic Dermatitis and Extremely High Total Serum IgE Levels Treated with High Doses of Omalizumab in Combination with Conventional Therapy

Maia Gotua, Nino Lomidze, Giorgi Shengelidze, Elene Kakabadze, Ketevan Kvaratskhelia, Nana Dolidze

CASE PRESENTATION

We present a case of 20 years old male with severe refractory atopic dermatitis (AD). The patient was diagnosed as having severe AD from childhood, sensitization to different dairy food products was revealed in early life. There was no positive family history of atopy or AD. From childhood, he was using permanent skincare products and was treated with topical corticosteroids, topical calcineurin inhibitors, and antihistamines. The patient was eliminating and avoiding exacerbating and trigger factors. Short courses of the systemic corticosteroids were used in case of severe exacerbations. The weight of a patient was 60 kg and height was 167 cm.

At 20 years of age, skin eruption was presented on the whole body including hands, face, flexural areas, anterior trunk, back, extremities, genitals with characteristic lichenified plaques, excoriations, oozing/crusts, erythema, swelling, xerosis, and a propensity for secondary staphylococcal infection (**Figs. 1A** to **D**). SCORing Atopic Dermatitis (SCORAD) index was 85, highly expressed pruritus (10 scores), with an extremely large effect on Dermatology Life Quality Index (DLQI)—25.

Patient's total serum immunoglobulin E (IgE) levels were extremely high—23, 210 kU/L, with high sensitization to environmental allergens—according to ImmunoCAP, Phadia results—sIgE Phadiatop >100 kUA/L Class 6 and food mixture sIgE fx5 (f1f2f3f4f13f14)—19.0 kUA/L Class 4. Molecular diagnostics (MADX) revealed clinically relevant very high sensitization to Timothy grass (Phl p1–32 kUA/L), Cypress (Cup a1–21 kUA/L), Ragweed (Amb a1–32 kUA/L), House Dust Mites (Der p1–29 kUA/L, Der p2–33 kUA/L, Der p23–32 kUA/L), and Cat (Fel d1–19 kUA/L). From food allergens, AD was triggered by Hazelnut (Cor a14–24 kUA/L). Other atopic conditions (asthma, allergic rhinitis, etc.) were not present. The count of eosinophils in the blood revealed 880 cells per microliter of blood (10%). Parasitosis, malignancies, and immunodeficiencies were excluded. Other parameters of the total blood count, erythrocyte sedimentation rate (ESR), liver, and kidney function tests, and C-reactive protein (CRP), were in the normal range.

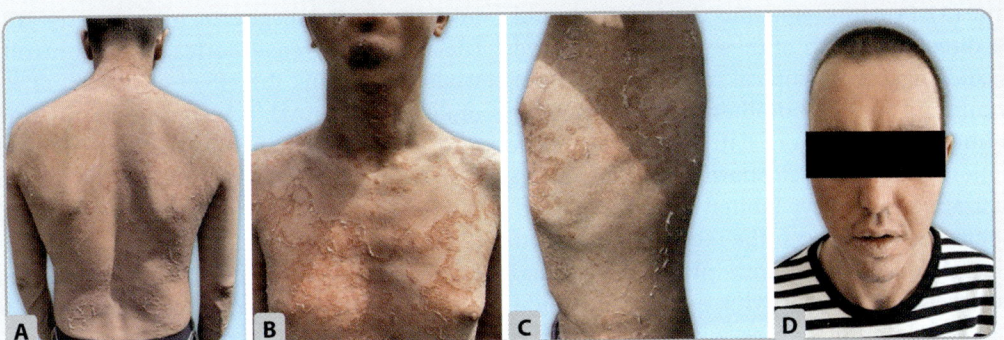

FIGS. 1A TO D: Skin eruptions on the body of the patient.

Because systemic immunosuppressive agents such as oral cyclosporine, methotrexate, and systemic corticosteroids all are associated with potentially serious adverse effects and require close clinical and laboratory monitoring, this kind of systemic therapy and phototherapy, as economically affordable therapies, was carefully discussed with the patient, as well as dupilumab treatment possibilities and costs.

The patient decided to leave a country and abroad was treated by omalizumab, with following scheme—four subsequent subcutaneous injections of 150 mg omalizumab in upper and lower extremities—600 mg/daily initially administered once in 4 weeks during 3 months and after in every 2 weeks during 5 months. Omalizumab was well tolerated without any immediate anaphylactic reaction, decreasing the severity of pruritus (symptom score of itching reduced to 3–4 scores), but for other symptoms of AD was not effective (SCORAD Index—75, DLQI—20). The skin lesions were a little bit better after omalizumab injections and then turned into the same condition. After 8 months of treatment, total IgE was 45,100 kU/L. When the treatment with omalizumab was stopped, after another 8 months, IgE was 38,550 kU/L.

DISCUSSION

In general, a high total serum IgE level is a biomarker for atopy and parasitosis. Very high [1,000 ≥ IgE (kU/L) <10,000] and extremely high total serum IgE levels (≥10,000) levels may raise suspicion for certain malignancies such as lymphoma and IgE myeloma. Elevated IgE levels may be seen in certain immunodeficiencies [hyper-IgE syndrome; Wiskott–Aldrich syndrome; immunodysregulation, polyendocrinopathy, enteropathy, X-linked (IPEX); Omenn syndrome; atypical complete DiGeorge syndrome; etc.].[1,2] The level of IgE and the degree of allergic sensitization are associated with severity of AD and contributed by abnormality of the skin barrier, a key feature of AD. A family history of atopy (eczema, asthma, or allergic rhinitis) and the loss-of-function mutations in the *Filaggrin* (*FLG*) gene, involved in the skin barrier function, are major risk factors for atopic dermatitis.[3] Elevated total IgE levels can be demonstrated in 80-85% of patients with AD, although the precise relationship between the elevated IgE levels and disease pathogenesis is unclear.[4] Children with very high IgE (>10,000 kU/L) are at greater risk for severe atopic dermatitis, sensitization to food and inhaled allergens, and anaphylaxis, compared with children with lesser elevations.[2-4]

Atopic dermatitis is a skin inflammatory disease with an increasing prevalence, affecting up to 20% of children and 2-5% of adults.[4-6] More than 80% of patients with AD have elevated IgE levels.[4,7,8] AD, as well as most forms of eczematous dermatitis, is characterized by three primary components—(1) Barrier failure, (2) Inflammatory immune response, and (3) Pruritus. Specific therapies should be directed at each of these components and include aggressive topical treatment with wet wraps and soaks, phototherapy, and systemic immunomodulators. Current treatments options, such as cyclosporine, methotrexate, or azathioprine, have limited effect on AD and numerous side effects. The recently introduced biologic dupilumab shows promising results; however, with conjunctivitis, as a prevalent side effect.[7-9] Unfortunately, because of the high cost of the drug, it was unaffordable for the patient.

Atopic dermatitis is a T-cell-driven complex inflammatory skin disease. The secretion of cytokines, involving not only particularly Th2, but also Th17 and Th22 cell subsets, provides a broad spectrum of potential targets. The new biological antibodies that target not only the Th2 cytokines—IL-4, IL-13, IL-31, as well as TSLP, IL-22 or IL-33, and innovative small molecules binding to the histamine-4 receptor, the phosphodiesterase-4, the aryl hydrocarbon receptor or downstream molecules such as Janus kinases have been published with promising results on symptoms and signs of atopic dermatitis.[5]

Omalizumab has been used for almost two decades, mainly in allergic asthma and chronic spontaneous urticaria for which it is highly beneficial.[2,3,6,9]

Systematic literature searches were performed in PubMed, Web of Science, Embase, and Clinicaltrials.gov to identify any study (case reports, case series, and controlled trials) evaluating the effect of treatment with omalizumab in AD.[10] According to this study, a total of 169 patients (79.0%) experienced a beneficial effect from treatment, ranging from little to complete response, whereas 45 patients (21.0%) reported no or negative effect from omalizumab treatment. Based on this study, omalizumab is a safe and well-tolerated treatment with some clinical benefits in AD patients. However, the lack of larger randomized controlled trials (RCTs) and possible publication bias limits the recommendation of omalizumab for use in clinical practice for AD. Newer and more effective treatments exist and should be prioritized.[10] Another authors are more critical and indicate that omalizumab has failed to produce benefit reproducibly and is not recommended for the treatment of adult eczemas.[7]

SUMMARY

High doses of omalizumab (1,200 mg subcutaneously per month) were safe and well tolerated without any anaphylactic reaction in a highly atopic patient with refractory severe AD and extremely high total serum IgE (>20,000 kU/L). It had a positive antipruritic effect, but no reaction to other symptoms of AD.

KEY MESSAGES

- Omalizumab, from point of view of anaphylactic reactions, is safe and well-tolerated treatment, even in high doses in a highly atopic patient with extremely high total serum IgE levels.
- Taking into account cost-effectiveness and clinical benefit of omalizumab on symptoms of AD, it is not recommended in case of severe refractory AD with extremely high total serum IgE levels; however, it has some positive effect on the reduction of itching.

REFERENCES

1. Ferastraoaru D, Bax HJ, Bergmann C, Capron M, Castells M, Dombrowicz D, et al. AllergoOncology: ultra-low IgE, a potential novel biomarker in cancer—a Position Paper of the European Academy of Allergy and Clinical Immunology (EAACI). Clin Transl Allergy. 2020;10:32.
2. Laske N, Bunikowski R, Niggemann B. Extraordinarily high serum IgE levels and consequences for atopic phenotypes. Ann Allergy Asthma Immunol. 2003;91:202-4.
3. Stokes J, Casale TB. (2020). The relationship between IgE and allergic disease. [online] Available from https://www.uptodate.com/contents/the-relationship-between-ige-and-allergic-disease. [Last accessed October, 2020].
4. Liu FT, Goodarzi H, Chen HY. IgE, mast cells, and eosinophils in atopic dermatitis. Clin Rev Allergy Immunol. 2011;41(3):298-310.
5. Deleanu D, Nedelea I. Biological therapies for atopic dermatitis: An update (Review). Exp Ther Med. 2019;17(2):1061-7.
6. Stokes J, Casale TB. (2020). The biology of IgE. [online] Available from https://www.uptodate.com/contents/the-biology-of-ige?source=related_link. [Last accessed October, 2020].
7. Berger TG. (2020). Evaluation and management of severe refractory atopic dermatitis (eczema) in adults. [online] Available from https://www.uptodate.com/contents/evaluation-and-management-of-severe-refractory-atopic-dermatitis-eczema-in-adults. [Last accessed October, 2020].
8. Holm JG, Agner T, Sand C, Thomsen SF. Omalizumab for atopic dermatitis: case series and a systematic review of the literature. Int J Dermatol. 2017;56(1):18-26.
9. Chia JC, Mydlarski PR. Dermatologic uses of omalizumabtitle. J Dermatolog Treat. 2017;28(4):332-7.
10. Holm JG, Thomsen SF. Omalizumab for atopic dermatitis: evidence for and against its use. G Ital Dermatol Venereol. 2019;154(4):480-7.

CASE 19

Atopic Dermatitis in Skin of Color

Kiran Godse, Kripa Ajmera, Gauri Godse, Anant Patil

CASE PRESENTATION

A 10-year-old Indian male presented with a 3-month history of hypopigmented lesion with mild itching and scaling, which started as a 1 × 1 cm in size and gradually progressed to 3 × 2 cm in size (**Fig. 1**). Patient revealed history of generalized dry skin and itching all over the body. The patient provided history of application of coconut oil as a measure to reduce the itching. It was useful in reducing itching, according to him.

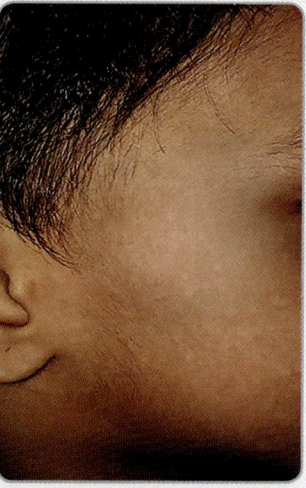

FIG. 1: Lesions on the skin.
Courtsey: Dr Kiran Nabar.

His mother provided history of frequent cold in patient during change of season. There was no history of loss of sensation on the patch. His mother and elder brother had history of bronchial asthma. Elder brother also had history of atopic rhinitis. There was no history of application of any topical agent.

On physical examination, a single ill-defined hypopigmented patch with scaling was observed on left cheek of the patient. Based on the clinical history and physical examination, the patient was diagnosed with atopic dermatitis showing a patch of pityriasis alba.

Patient was treated with emollient all over the body. Topical 0.1% tacrolimus ointment was prescribed for application on the localized skin patch.

The patient started showing improvement in 4 weeks and was continued on emollients.

DISCUSSION

Atopic dermatitis is believed to be six times more common in black children than white children.[1] Diagnosing atopic dermatitis in skin of color patients can be a challenge because erythema can be harder to identify in skin with darker tones, meaning that atopic dermatitis may be missed or undertreated in deeply pigmented adolescents.[1]

Pityriasis alba, benign dermatosis, is commonly seen in children and shows an ill-defined hypopigmented macule or patch on face. It is included in one of the minor criteria of atopic dermatitis given by Hanifin and Rajka in 1980, which also includes other forms of eczema such as cheilitis, nipple eczema, facial pallor/erythema, orbital darkening, and hand and foot eczema. Out of these, pityriasis alba is difficult to be appreciated in patients with Fitzpatrick skin type I, II, and III. Patients with skin of color show classic pityriasis alba. It has a prevalence of 1.9–5.2% and is more often seen among the people belonging to the darkly pigmented races.[2] Hence, it is imperative to examine for other cutaneous signs of atopic dermatitis such as xerosis, Dennie–Morgan lines, palmar hyperlinearity, and atopic dirty neck.

Pityriasis means fine scale and alba means pale color or hypopigmentation. These lesions may be mildly erythematous and over time become hypopigmented. It is difficult to appreciate the erythema in skin of color. Hypopigmented lesions are appreciated well in such patients. These lesions are usually few in number measuring 0.5–5 cm in size. They are most commonly seen on face especially on cheeks, arms, and upper trunk. Sun exposure may accentuate the lesion. These scales usually increase in winter due to dry air, and lesions become more accentuated in spring and summer because of sun exposure and darkening of the surrounding skin. It has noncontagious and noninfectious etiology. Children with pityriasis alba shows history of atopy. These lesions usually resolve spontaneously. Classically, histopathology shows reduced melanin production in the stratum basale. The number of active melanocytes and size remains normal.

These lesions have to be differentiated from leprosy, postinflammatory hypopigmentation, fungal infection such as tinea versicolor, tinea corporis, vitiligo, nevus depigmentosus, psoriasis, seborrhea, ash leaf macules of tuberous sclerosis, mycosis fungoides, post-steroid hypopigmentation, and hypopigmented polymorphous light eruption.

If the diagnosis is uncertain, several diagnostic procedures may be useful. On examination with a Wood's lamp, the lesions of pityriasis alba may be accentuated but are nonfluorescent. This finding is in contrast to vitiligo, which will fluoresce more brightly and have edges with sharper demarcation. Potassium hydroxide (KOH) preparation of a skin scraping is negative for fungal elements. This result is in contrast to tinea versicolor or tinea corporis, which is positive for fungal elements. Skin biopsy is usually not necessary, but when performed, it can distinguish pityriasis alba from mycosis fungoides.[3,4]

Lesions of pityriasis alba are usually self-resolving, which usually take about a month to few years. Low-potent topical corticosteroid such as 1% hydrocortisone cream or ointment can be used to reduce erythema and pruritus. Mild emollient such as petroleum jelly and cream may reduce scaling. Sun protection with broad-spectrum sunscreen, wide-brim hat, and long-sleeve clothes protect the skin from sun burning and decrease the darkening around the skin and improve the cosmetic appearance. Patient can also be treated with topical calcineurin inhibitor, calcitriol, or topical vitamin D analog. Psoralen plus ultraviolet A (PUVA) photochemotherapy and targeted phototherapy with 308-nm excimer laser is also used.

Adolescents with atopic dermatitis should use moisturizers containing ceramide.[5] Patients with skin of color often experience postinflammatory hyperpigmentation in AD and acne or hypopigmentation from inflammatory dermatoses including AD.[6,7]

A pigmentary variant of pityriasis alba is more commonly seen in patients with darker skin such as South Africa and Middle East. These present as central zone of bluish hyperpigmentation surrounded by hypopigmented halo. It is usually associated with fungal infection. It is postulated that AD has a greater impact on quality of life (QOL) in children with skin of color, resulting in the increased number of school absences in this population.[5]

CONCLUSION

Patients with atopic dermatitis have a minor criterion of pityriasis alba, which presents with hypopigmented macule or patch with mild scaling on face in children and this is usually seen on face. These lesions are difficult to appreciate in fair-skinned individual.

KEY MESSAGES

- Patients who present with hypopigmented macule or patch on the face should be differentiated from pityriasis alba, leprosy, pityriasis versicolor, and postinflammatory hypopigmentation.
- Given the social and emotional impact of atopic dermatitis on patients with skin of color, it is necessary to treat the condition appropriately.

REFERENCES

1. Ben-Gashir MA, Hay RJ. Reliance on erythema scores may mask severe atopic dermatitis in black children compared with their white counterparts. Br J Dermatol. 2002;147(5):920-5.
2. Miazek N, Michalek I, Pawlowska-Kisiel M, Olszewska M, Rudnicka L. Pityriasis alba—Common disease, enigmatic entity: Up-to-date review of the literature. Pediatr Dermatol. 2015;32(6):786-91.
3. Jadotte YT, Janniger CK. Pityriasis alba revisited: perspectives on an enigmatic disorder of childhood. Cutis. 2011;87(2):66-72.
4. Gameiro A, Gouveia M, Tellechea Ó, Moreno A. Childhood hypopigmented mycosis fungoides: a commonly delayed diagnosis. BMJ Case Rep. 2014;23:2014.
5. Wan J, Margolis DJ, Mitra N, Hoffstad OJ, Takeshita J. Racial and ethnic differences in atopic dermatitis-related school absences among US children. JAMA Dermatol. 2019;155:973-75.
6. Vachiramon V, Tey HL, Thompson AE. Atopic dermatitis in African American children: addressing unmet needs of a common disease. Pediatr Dermatol. 2012;29:395-402.
7. Heath CR. Managing postinflammatory hyperpigmentation in pediatric patients with skin of color. Cutis. 2018;102:71-3.

CASE 20

Herbal Preparations Causing Irritation in a Patient with Atopic Dermatitis: A Case Report

Tejaswini Shekhar Sharma, Gauri Godse, Anant Patil, Feroz K

CASE PRESENTATION

A 30-year-old female, homemaker, known case of atopic dermatitis, presented with itchy red lesions over her whole body since 3 months. Lesions first started to involve flexures of hand, back, lower limb, and further involved inframammary region.

She was previously treated with multiple topical steroid creams and antiallergic oral medications but with temporary relief.

The patient had history of using herbal preparations such as neem and tulsi leaves to relieve itching as advised by someone. Use of these preparations led to worsening of lesion and extensive itching after their application.

There was no history of diabetes mellitus, hypertension, ischemic heart disease, atopy, asthma, or any other comorbidity. The patient also did not have past history of similar illness or relevant family history.

On clinical examination, multiple, ill-defined, symmetrical, erythematous papules coalescing to form plaques with excoriation involving flexural areas, back trunk, inframammary region, thighs, and buttocks were seen (**Figs. 1A** to **D**).

The patient was counseled regarding the chronic nature of disease and was advised to stop use of herbal creams. The patient was started on oral prednisolone 20 mg, hydroxyzine 10 mg, and fusidic acid plus betamethasone cream twice daily for 7 days. Later, patient was advised to use emollient immediately after bath and apply mometasone furoate (0.1%) at night. Patient showed significant improvement in 4 weeks.

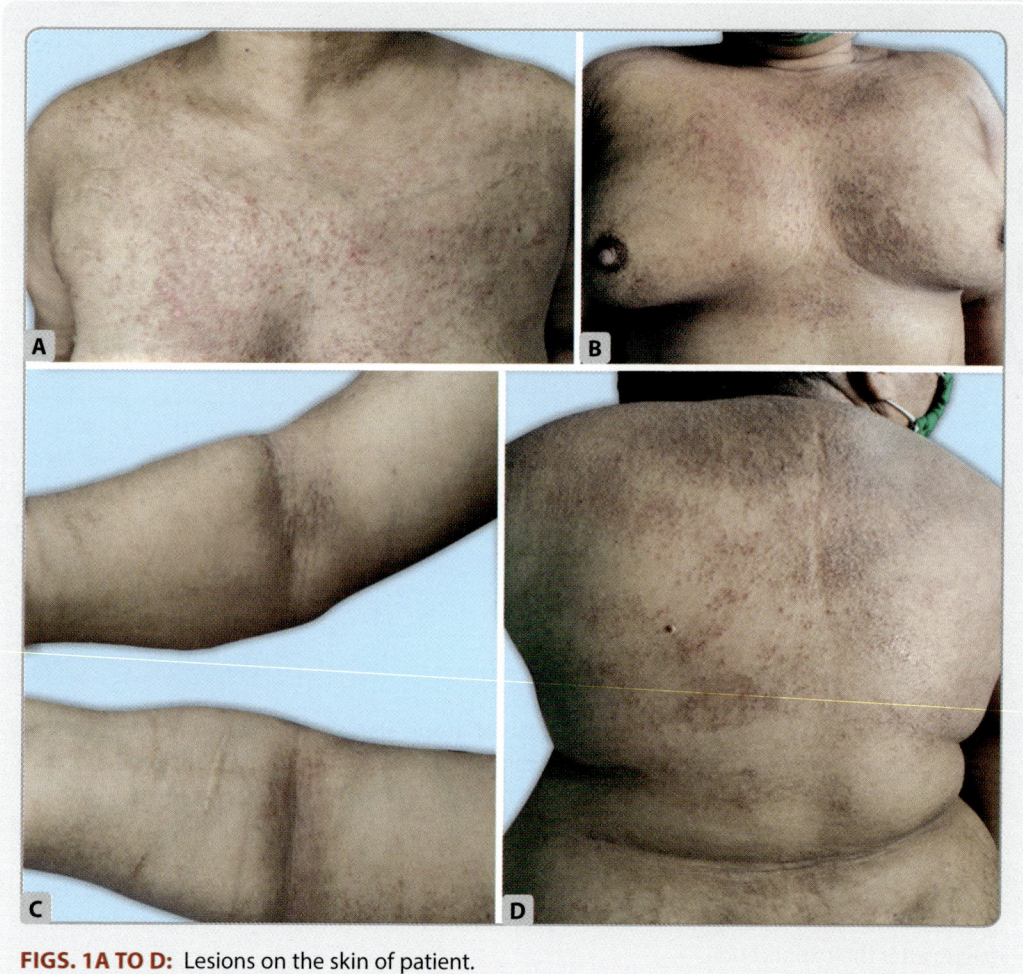

FIGS. 1A TO D: Lesions on the skin of patient.

DISCUSSION

Use of plant-derived preparation is not uncommon for the treatment for several diseases. Some of the examples of plants with health benefits include *Achyranthes aspera, Allium cepa, Allium sativum, Aloe vera, Azadirachta indica* (known as neem), *Bauhinia variegata*, etc.[1] Herbal therapies, e.g., traditional Chinese herbal therapy, have been reported to be useful in the treatment of atopic eczema.[2] Suppression of inflammatory mediators release from mast cell is suggested to play a role in atopic eczema.[3]

Usage of herbal preparations is popular and has grown both in developed and developing countries[4] due to some documented benefits and few perceived by the patients.[5] Neem has been suggested to have diverse utility.[6]

Although herbal preparations are commonly used, many products lack strong evidence derived by large well-designed clinical trials.[4]

Moreover, against the traditional belief that these preparations are free from side effects, some patients can develop adverse events with herbal preparations.[7] Most patients using herbal preparations may not be aware about their potential in resulting adverse events.[8]

As some patients use herbal preparations for treatment of skin diseases, dermatologists should also be aware about its possible adverse effects. Adverse effects such as allergic reactions and photosensitization are possible with herbal remedies. Some preparations may contain chemicals such as arsenic or mercury or other products causing skin reactions.[9]

We present a case of chronic/chronically relapsing hypersensitive reaction with itching as predominant feature.

Neem (*Azadirachta indica*) being an antioxidant has role in scavenging of free radicals. Neem has anti-inflammatory activity due to regulation of proinflammatory enzyme activities.[10] Use of holy basil (tulsi) is also common in India.[11]

In India, herbal preparations, both topical and oral, are often used by the patients for treatment of chronic skin diseases. The use of herbal preparations is increasing day-by-day as they have been reported to reduce eczema like skin lesions but in few patients, like this case, may show exacerbation of disease on application. Consequently, they have potential adverse effects such as skin eruption. Neem has therapeutic implications and has been traditionally used worldwide, but in few cases of atopic dermatitis, it can result in irritant reaction.

CONCLUSION

Herbal preparation may cause irritant reaction in some patients with atopic dermatitis. Patients should be educated about the potential of adverse effects with herbal products. Before using any product, dermatologists should ensure its proof of safety and efficacy in skin condition.

KEY MESSAGES

- Herbal preparations are perceived safe by the general population; however, they may be associated with side effects in some patients with atopic dermatitis.
- Dermatologists should be aware about potential of causing adverse effects with use of herbal preparations.

REFERENCES

1. Tabassum N, Hamdani M. Plants used to treat skin diseases. Pharmacogn Rev. 2014;8(15):52-60.
2. Latchman Y, Whittle B, Rustin M, Atherton DJ, Brostoff J. The efficacy of traditional Chinese herbal therapy in atopic eczema. Int Arch Allergy Immunol. 1994;104(3):222-6.
3. Chan BCL, Hon KLE, Leung PC, Sam SW, Fung KP, Lee MYH, et al. Traditional Chinese medicine for atopic eczema: PentaHerbs formula suppresses inflammatory mediators release from mast cells. J Ethnopharmacol. 2008;120(1):85-91.
4. Calixto JB. Efficacy, safety, quality control, marketing and regulatory guidelines for herbal medicines (phytotherapeutic agents). Braz J Med Biol Res. 2000;33(2):179-89.
5. Kaur J, Kaur S, Mahajan A. Herbal medicines: Possible risks and benefits. Am J Phytomed Clin Therap. 2013;2:226-39.
6. Brahmachari G. Neem—an omnipotent plant: A retrospection. Chem Bio Chem. 2004;5(4):408-21.
7. Faghihi G, Radan M. Side effects of herbal drugs used in dermatologic disorders. J Cosm Dermatol Sci App. 2011;1:1-3.
8. Gari M, Majhee L, Kumari K. Herbal drug-induced adverse drug reaction: A case report. Asian J Pharm Clin Re. 2018;1:9-11.
9. Ernst E. Adverse effects of herbal drugs in dermatology. Brit J Dermatol. 2000;143:923-29.
10. Alzohairy MA. Therapeutics role of *Azadirachta indica* (Neem) and their active constituents in diseases prevention and treatment. Evid Based Complement Alternat Med. 2016;2016:7382506.
11. Kumar S, Swarankar V, Sharma S, Baldi A. Herbal cosmetics: Used for skin and hair. Inventi Rapid: Cosmeceuticals. 2012;4:1-7.

SECTION 2

Interesting Cases: Pruritus

CASE 1

Long-term Efficacy and Safety of Dupilumab in Prurigo Nodularis: A Case Report

Germiniasi F, Tavecchio S, L Angileri, Berti E, Ferrucci S

CASE PRESENTATION

A 46-year-old woman complained of intensely pruritic papules and nodules predominantly on her legs for 4 years. Pathology showed psoriasiform epidermal hyperplasia with hypergranulosis, overlying compact hyperkeratosis and dermal perivascular lymphocytic infiltrate, consistent with a diagnosis of prurigo nodularis (PN). Indirect immunofluorescence (IIF) ruled out an autoimmune bullous disorder. The patient referred a good general health and blood tests were within normal limits, included eosinophil count and total serum immunoglobulin E (IgE). Skin prick tests and patch tests were negative.

Over a 3-year period, the patient was treated with several cycles of topical and systemic corticosteroids, systemic antihistamines, topical calcineurin inhibitor ointments, and narrow-band ultraviolet B therapy. The pruritus remained poorly controlled and the patient had very poor quality of life. A psychiatric evaluation was also recommended. As a final attempt, the patient was treated with cyclosporine 2–3 mg/kg/die for further 3 years uninterruptedly, ultimately resulting in good control of the disease, despite kidney failure and blood hypertension onset.

Six months after stopping the therapy, pruritus worsened again and the patient came to our attention. The skin examination showed excoriated papules and nodules extended over the extensor surface of arms and trunk, along with very intense pruritus and dry skin (**Fig. 1**). Methotrexate (maximum dose 15 mg/week) failed to provide any improvement to the lesions, and was stopped after 1 year because of nausea and diarrhea. Based on blood test and blood pressure within normal limits, the patient underwent another cycle of cyclosporine 2 mg/kg/die with gradual improvement of pruritus and smoothing of nodular lesions. Two years later, cyclosporine was gradually tapered and, eventually, discontinued. Treatment with tricyclic antidepressants such as amitriptyline and antiepileptic drugs such as gabapentin and pregabalin was started without any clinical improvement. Azathioprine (50 mg/die) did not give any benefit too. Clinical findings slightly worsened with numerous excoriated nodules spread throughout limbs and trunk.

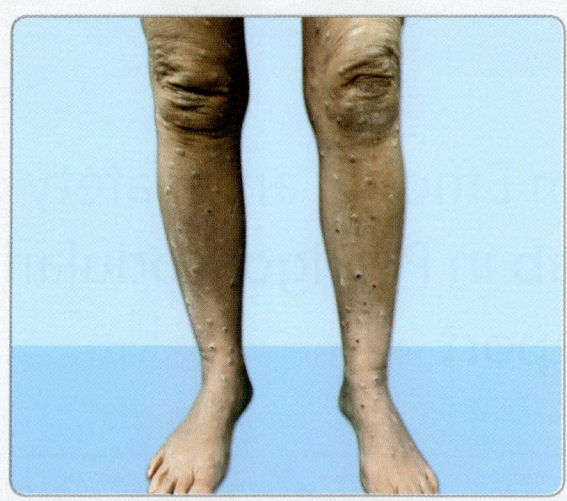

FIG. 1: Skin lesions before initiating dupilumab.

TABLE 1: Physician-reported and patient-reported outcomes at baseline (T0), week 4 (T4), week 16 (T16), week 32 (T32), week 52 (T52) and week 64 (T64) after dupilumab starting.

						HADS	
	EASI	DLQI	NRS-itch	VAS-sleep	POEM	D	A
T0	42	28	10	10	28	10	14
T4	28	18	6	6	14	9	9
T16	5	18	2	0	12	7	8
T32	3	18	1	0	12	8	9
T52	3	11	1	0	11	7	7
T64	0	2	0	0	4	3	4

(A: anxiety; D: depression; DLQI; Dermatology Life Quality Index; EASI: Eczema Area and Severity Index; HADS: Hospital Anxiety and Depression Scale; NRS: Numerical Rating Scale; POEM: Patient-oriented Eczema Measure; VAS: Visual Analog Sleep)

Finally, the patient, at age of 57, received her first dose of off-label dupilumab 600 mg administered subcutaneously by the clinician. The loading dose was followed by dupilumab 300 mg, self-administered every 2 weeks, associated with topical corticosteroid medications and emollients. Because no standardized rating scale for PN exists, clinical response was evaluated using atopic dermatitis scores.[1] Before and regularly after treatment, disease severity was assessed through the Eczema Area and Severity Index (EASI, range 0–72)—considering the extension and severity of prurigo lesions instead of eczema. Quality of life was evaluated by some patient-reported outcomes including the Italian version of Dermatology Life Quality Index (DLQI, range 0–30) questionnaire, Patient-oriented Eczema Measure (POEM, range 0–28), Hospital Anxiety and Depression Scale (HADS, range 0–21), Peak Pruritus Numerical Rating Scale (NRS-itch, range 0–10), and Visual Analog Sleep (VAS-sleep, range 0–10). As shown in **Table 1**, after 1 month of treatment (T4), the patient was already showing considerable improvement—the EASI score, which was 42 at baseline, dropped to 28, the DLQI score dropped from 28 at baseline to 18 and the POEM score dropped from 28 to 14. NRS-itch and VAS-sleep scores, which were 10 at baseline, dropped to 6. Similarly, HADS-anxiety at baseline was 14 and dropped to 9 while HADS-depression dropped from 10 to 9. The improvement was maintained over time (**Table 1**). At 16-month follow-up (T64), pruritus disappeared (NRS-itch 0), quality of sleeping drastically improved (VAS-sleep: 0) as well as quality of life (DLQI: 4, HADS-anxiety: 4, HADS-depression: 3), and extension and severity of skin lesions (EASI: 0). No adverse events were reported. The patient is currently on therapy with dupilumab associated with daily emollients and topical corticosteroid upon request, while the antidepressants have been discontinued. Skin examination now shows only scars and pigmentation (**Fig. 2**).

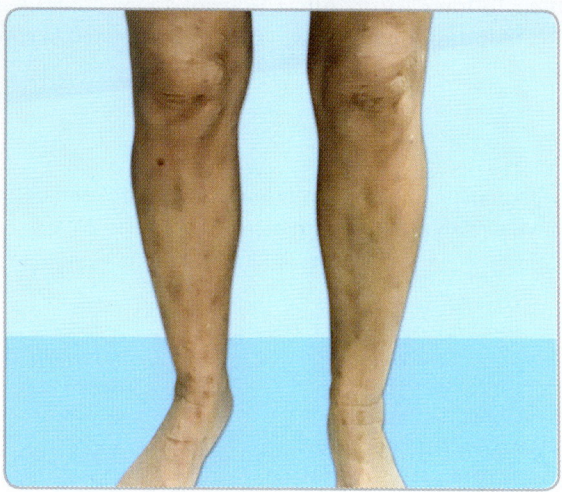

FIG. 2: Skin examination after dupilumab treatment.

DISCUSSION

In this case report, we present a patient with recalcitrant prurigo nodularis (PN) who failed many therapies. In particular, the severe pruritus caused sleep disturbance, work productivity impairment, anxiety, and depression. PN is a disease characterized by papulonodules as consequence of chronic scratching of the skin due to intense pruritus.[2] Lesions typically occur in areas easily accessible to the patient (the extensor surfaces of arms, back, chest, and face).

This condition is difficult to treat and treatment response is often frustrating. The absence of approved therapies for PN allows clinicians to use numerous different therapies that often cause significant side effects without any improvement to the disease.[2]

The PN pathophysiology is hypothesized and to be mediated by a Th2 helper cell response, similar to that seen in atopic dermatitis (AD). Moreover, recent evidence has suggested that, apart from histamine, several mediators and signaling pathways are involved in the pathogenesis of pruritus, in particular interleukin (IL)-4 and IL-13, the hallmark of AD.[3,4] Therefore, treatment of PN with anti IL-4 and IL-13 biologic therapies would be expected to elicit a therapeutic response. Furthermore, IL-4 and IL-13 are the main upstream drivers in the Th2 pathways that modulate numerous downstream targets, such as IL-5 and IL-31.[4,5]

Another approach relates the effectiveness of dupilumab to the fact that PN represents a clinical manifestation of an underlying AD.[2] However, we can rule out such relation, since that patient did not show any sign of atopic skin diathesis.

CONCLUSION

The present case, which follows up to our previous cases,[6] suggests that dupilumab may be a useful and effective therapy for PN since that patient experienced reduction of pruritus symptoms and subsequent improvement in prurigo lesions within 6 months of treatment, leading to an increase in quality of life. Its effectiveness seems to be independent from an underlying atopy.

The response following dupilumab treatment in this patient is encouraging and raises the hope of a new potential therapy of PN. Further studies are needed to confirm this prospect.

KEY MESSAGE

- The treatment of PN with dupilumab significantly improves pruritus and decreases the extension and the size of the lesions already after 1 month of treatment.

REFERENCES

1. Ferrucci S, Casazza G, Angileri L, Tavecchio F, Germiniasi F, Berti E, et al. Clinical response and quality of life in patients with severe atopic dermatitis treated with dupilumab: A single-center real-life experience. J Clin Med. 2020;9(3):791.
2. Zeidler C, Yosipovitch G, Ständer S. Prurigo nodularis and its management. Dermatol Clin. 2018;36(3):189-97.
3. Fukushi S, Yamasaki K, Aiba S. Nuclear localization of activated STAT6 and STAT3 in epidermis of prurigo nodularis. Br J Dermatol. 2011;165(5):990-6.
4. Pavlis J, Yosipovitch G. Management of Itch in Atopic Dermatitis. Am J Clin Dermatol. 2018;19(3): 319-32.
5. Zhai LL, Savage KT, Qiu CC, Jin A, Valdes-Rodriguez R, Mollanazar NK. Chronic Pruritus Responding to Dupilumab-A Case Series. Medicines (Basel). 2019;6(3):72.
6. Ferrucci S, Tavecchio S, Berti E, Angileri L. Dupilumab and prurigo nodularis-like phenotype in atopic dermatitis: Our experience of efficacy. J Dermatol Treat. 2019;1-2.

CASE 2

Generalized Purpuric Macules with Intense Pruritus: A Single Case Report

*Chuda Rujitharanawong, Nuttagarn Jantanapornchai, Charussri Leeyaphan,
Penvadee Pattanaprichakul, Kanokvalai Kulthanan*

CASE PRESENTATION

A 73-year-old Thai female presented with a 3-month history of generalized intense itching and progressive skin lesions. Her underlying diseases included hypertension and dyslipidemia. Her regular medications were aspirin, telmisartan, manidipine, hydrochlorothiazide, and simvastatin. She denied changing any medications prior to developing the rash. She and her family were otherwise healthy.

Physical examination revealed numerous generalized discrete purpuric macules and excoriated papules located predominantly on the buttocks and both upper thighs, and both of these clinical manifestations are associated with intense pruritus (**Fig. 1**).

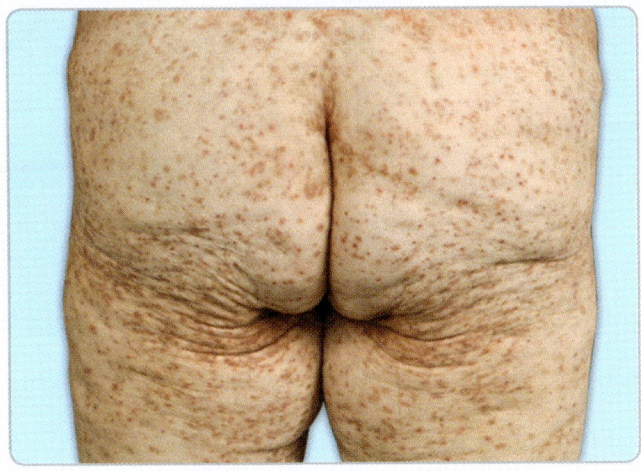

FIG. 1: A 73-year-old Thai female presented with numerous generalized itchy discrete purpuric macules and excoriated papules located predominantly on the buttocks and both upper thighs.

Skin biopsy from the left thigh revealed leukocytoclastic vasculitis (**Fig. 2**).

During the period between the biopsy and the biopsy result, she developed new lesions on both axillae and finger webs. Skin scraping revealed mites, eggs, and feces of *Sarcoptes scabiei* (**Fig. 3**).

She was diagnosed as scabiasis with vasculitis reaction, and she was treated with oral ivermectin 12 mg per week for 2 consecutive weeks together with topical 25% benzyl benzoate. After 2 weeks of treatment, her itchy symptom and skin lesions were markedly improved, and repeated skin scraping examination was negative.

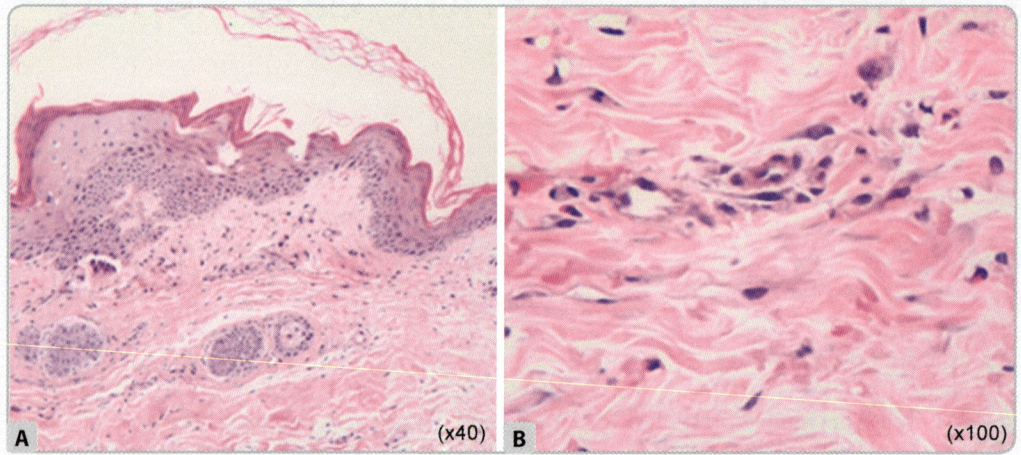

FIGS. 2A AND B: Skin biopsy from her left thigh revealed leukocytoclastic vasculitis.

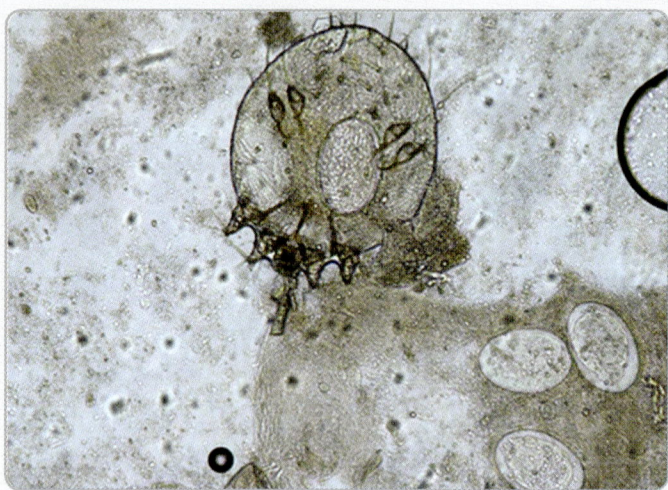

FIG. 3: Microscopic examination of skin scraping from her left palm revealed mites and eggs of *Sarcoptes scabiei*.

DISCUSSION

Scabies is a skin infection that is caused by *Sarcoptes scabies* variety *hominis*.[1] Host immune reaction to the burrowed mites and theirs byproducts is likely due to itchy symptom and scabietic skin lesion.[2] Onset in a host with first-time infestation was reported to occur after 2-6 weeks,[3] and reinfestation can provoke symptoms within 24-48 hours.[4] The typical manifestations include papules, vesicles, pustules, and nodules that are normally located at the interdigital web spaces, axillary folds, periumbilical area, and genital area.[2] According to the 2020 International Alliance for the Control of Scabies (IACS) criteria, two history features (i.e., itch and close contact with someone who has scabies) are mandatory for a diagnosis of scabies in patients with atypical lesions or atypical distribution.[1] However, this patient presented with atypical itchy vasculitic skin lesions without history of close contact with someone who has scabies.

Scabietic vasculitis is a rare, but previously reported condition.[5-7] Leukocytoclastic vasculitis is a hypersensitivity reaction to scabies infection. The proposed mechanism of this reaction is humoral immune response that develops due to circulating antigen-antibody immune complexes to antigenic debris in the blood from pruritic excoriations.[7,8] Onset of pruritus is normally 1-8 months before the development of purpuric lesions.[8] Patients with scabietic vasculitis can be healthy or immunocompromised patients, and the average age was reported to be 65 years.[7]

In generalized and crusted scabies, combination of oral ivermectin and a topical scabicide is recommended.[9] Oral ivermectin 200 μg/kg per week for 2 consecutive weeks is a highly effective treatment with a good safely profile. Permethrin 5% has been widely used due to its high efficacy, good patient tolerance, and low toxicity. Benzyl benzoate 25% lotion has good efficacy, but it frequently causes skin irritation. Precipitated sulfur 5-10% has been effectively used in young children and pregnant women. Gamma benzene hexachloride is no longer used due to its neurotoxic effect. Close contact persons, including family members and sexual partners, should be treated simultaneously to avoid reinfestation and transmission.[9] Clothing and bedding should be sanitized by washing in hot water or sealing in a plastic bag for at least 72 hours. Symptomatic treatment for pruritus, including antihistamines or steroids, may be considered. Secondary bacterial infection is a common complication that requires appropriate treatment.

CONCLUSION

Patients with scabies infection can present with vasculitis, which is a reaction to scabietic debris in circulating blood that results from pruritic excoriations. Intense pruritus symptom is a useful clue for a diagnosis of scabies infection in patients with atypical presentation.

KEY MESSAGE

- Patients who present with cutaneous vasculitis and intense pruritus should be investigated scabies infection.

REFERENCES

1. Engelman D, Yoshizumi J, Hay RJ, Osti M, Micali G, Norton S, et al. The 2020 IACS Consensus Criteria for the Diagnosis of Scabies. Br J Dermatol. 2020. Online ahead of print.
2. McCarthy JS, Kemp DJ, Walton SF, Currie BJ. Scabies: more than just an irritation. Postgrad Med J. 2004;80(945):382-7.
3. Kang S, Amagai M, Bruckner AL, Enk AH, Margolis DJ, McMichael AJ, et al. Fitzpatrick's Dermatology, 9th edition. New York: McGraw-Hill Education; 2018.
4. Maghrabi MM, Lum S, Joba AT, Meier MJ, Holmbeck RJ, Kennedy K. Norwegian crusted scabies: an unusual case presentation. J Foot Ankle Surg. 2014;53:62-6.
5. Valks R, Buezo GF, Dauden E. Scabies and leukocytoclastic vasculitis in an HIV-seropositive man. Int J Dermatol. 1996;35:605-6.
6. Nishihara K, Shiraishi K, Sayama K. Leukocytoclastic vasculitis associated with crusted scabies. Eur J Dermatol. 2018;28:242-3.
7. Clevy C, Brajon D, Combes E, Benzaquen M, Dales JP, Koeppel MC, et al. Scabietic vasculitis: Report of 2 cases. Ann Dermatol Venereol. 2017;144:349-55.
8. Cabrera R, Agar A, Dahl MV. The immunology of scabies. Semin Dermatol. 1993;12:15-21.
9. McGoldrick M. Scabies Infestation. Home Healthc Now. 2015;33:503-4.

CASE 3

Importance of Dietary History in the Presence of a Biopsy Suggestive of Urticarial Vasculitis

Iman Nasr, Humaid A Al Wahshi, Shamsa H Al Maawali, Ethar Said Mohamed Al Hajri

CASE PRESENTATION

A 23-year-old lady was referred to the adult immunology clinic in September 2019, for evaluation of itchy urticarial lesions of the upper limbs and trunk (**Fig. 1**). She reported that since the beginning of May 2019, around the end of the 2nd week of following a strict ketogenic diet, very itchy maculopapular skin rashes appeared after an hour of eating cookies made of coconut flour. The rashes initially started on bilateral arm flexors that lasted for few days then subsided. She was not aware of the cause and continued the same diet. Few days later, they appeared on the lower back and spread proximally over the back, slightly on abdomen and chest. For symptomatic relief, the patient bought over the counter 4 mg of chlorphenamine maleate from the pharmacy to be taken every 4–6 hours, unfortunately the lesions did not improve but worsened. The rashes lasted for roughly a week then began to resolve gradually leaving hyperpigmentation. The patient stopped the ketogenic diet and followed a normal diet for 3 months during which the rash never came back. However, the rash reappeared 3 days after restarting the ketogenic diet around the mid of August 2019; an hour after, she accidentally had coconut milk. She developed itchy maculopapular skin rash over her body. She was referred to the dermatology department where she was diagnosed with urticaria. She had tried cetirizine 10 mg once daily for 30 days with no effect, mometasone furoate (cream 0.1%) once daily as well as fexofenadine 180 mg once daily for 14 days also with no effect. She had prednisolone 30 mg once daily for 3 days and thought was effective; however, the rashes were in their last stage of resolution when she had the prednisolone. She also reported that she noticed that the rashes were also triggered by milk and its derivatives, so she stopped both coconut and dairy products. The symptoms were also exacerbated by warm weather, hot shower, and exercise. After repeated episodes, the patient presented to the immunologist and allergist for further investigation. She had no symptoms to suggest autoimmunity. She had no angioedema, respiratory symptoms, fever, or constitutional symptoms. No joint pains or change in bowel habit. She had no family history of autoimmunity nor similar complaints. She had blood and urine tests done as well as skin biopsy taken from two active lesions. The patient continued

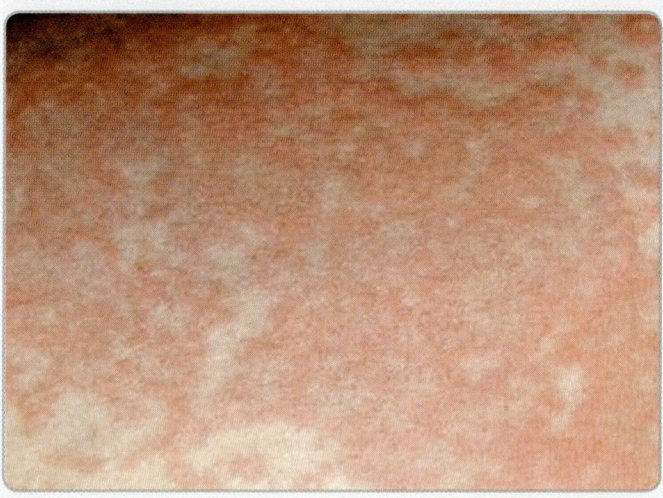

FIG. 1: Rash of prurigo pigmentosa.

the ketogenic diet for 2 months with a total of 3–4 episodes of skin rashes each lasting around a week. She had prednisolone 30 mg once daily for 3 days at the onset of the rash for the 2nd time, but no improvement occurred. While the patient was waiting for the results of the skin biopsy and blood workup, she decided to do a diet modification by stopping the ketogenic diet and increase the amount of carbohydrate taken. The rash never occurred since.

Examination revealed a well-built lady, blood pressure was normal 126/78 mm Hg, pulse was 82 bpm, oxygen saturation was 99% on room air, and she had active erythematous papules with hyperpigmented lesions over the upper limbs, chest, and back.

Skin biopsy was done (**Figs. 2A** to **D**), which showed skin with epidermis showing mild hyperkeratosis, mild spongiosis, and mild interphase change. The superficial dermis is mildly edematous, and shows moderate perivascular infiltration dominated by lymphocytes with few histiocytes and occasional neutrophils. Toluidine blue highlights occasional mast cells. Immunofluorescent staining was positive for immunoglobulin A (IgA) and C3. Features are compatible with lymphocytic vasculitis.

Blood workup showed normal full blood count, kidney, and liver functions. Antinuclear antibody (ANA) was 1:100, and extractable nuclear antibody (ENA) was positive for polymyositis/scleroderma (PM/Scl); anti-double-stranded DNA. Urine protein–creatinine ratio was negative, normal C-reactive protein (CRP), erythrocyte sedimentation rate (ESR), and complements. Hepatitis B and C and HIV were negative so were anticitrullinated peptide and rheumatoid factor. Cryoglobulin was negative and so was antineutrophil cytoplasmic antibody (ANCA). Thyroid peroxidase antibody (TPO) was positive—74.6, but normal thyroid function. In view of the suspicion of lesions occurring within an hour of consuming coconut and cow milk, specific immunoglobulin E (IgE) to coconut and cow milk was negative. Total IgE was slightly raised 246 [normal range (NR) 0–100], IgG slightly raised 20.9 (5.4–18.22), normal IgA and IgM.

The initial diagnosis based on skin biopsy was urticarial vasculitis and she was referred to the rheumatology team for further evaluation. Their impression was vasculitis likely secondary to a viral insult but unlikely due to connective tissue disease in the absence of other symptoms.

CASE 3 Importance of Dietary History in the Presence of a Biopsy Suggestive of Urticarial Vasculitis

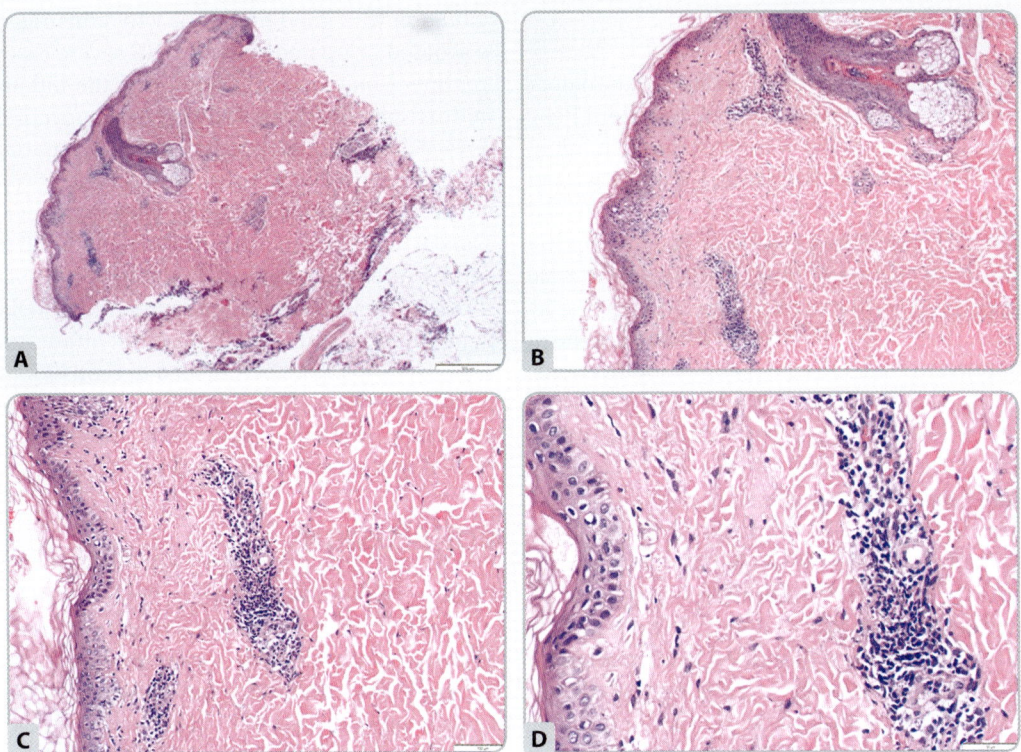

FIGS. 2A TO D: Histopathological features of prurigo pigmentosa.

She was planned to be treated with tapering doses of steroids; however, the patient was worried about the side effects of prednisolone and opted not to take it. She also decided to stop the ketogenic diet. On follow-up, 2 months later, the patient had no further recurrence in her symptoms since stopping the ketogenic diet and remains asymptomatic 6 months later to date. She could drink cow milk and eat coconut many times without symptoms and still has no symptoms to suggest autoimmune disease. The final diagnosis was revised as self-limiting prurigo pigmentosa (PP) especially with the absence of features to suggest autoimmune disease and the disappearance of symptoms on stopping the ketogenic diet without the need to be on oral steroids and as a result the positive ENA was thought to be a false-positive result. She was advised to repeat the serology after 1 year and report any new symptoms that may appear.

Erythematous papules were intensely itchy and distributed symmetrically over the neck, chest, abdomen, upper, and lower limbs lasting around a week and healing with hyperpigmentation.

These stained with hematoxylin and eosin with magnification 40×, 100×, 200×, 400×, respectively. Skin biopsy shows skin with epidermis showing mild hyperkeratosis, mild spongiosis, and mild interphase change. The superficial dermis is mildly edematous, shows moderate perivascular infiltration dominated by lymphocytes with few histiocytes and occasional neutrophils. Toluidine blue highlights occasional mast cells. Immunofluorescent staining was positive for immunoglobulin A (IgA) and C3. Features are compatible with lymphocytic vasculitis.

DISCUSSION

Prurigo pigmentosa (PP) is a rare inflammatory skin condition characterized by recurrent itchy red papules that heal with hyperpigmentation. It is also known as Nagashima disease named after the person who described it and published in April, 1978.[1] The cause is unknown, but the condition has been described in many case reports linked to strict ketogenic diet giving its name "Keto rash."[2-4] Onset of PP has also been reported to coincide with dietary modifications, fasting, weight loss, and diabetes mellitus.[5-9]

The lesions of PP occur on the trunk, upper and lower limbs, and the nape of the neck. There were no reports of mucosal involvement.[6] Early in the course, the lesions are typically erythematous and intensely itchy that resolve (usually without treatment) into pigmented macules. Lesions last for approximately 1 week. The histopathology described in the literature showed superficial perivascular and interstitial infiltrate of neutrophils early in the disease. Later on, patchy lymphocytic infiltrate and necrosis of numerous keratinocytes follow. Late lesions show lymphocytic infiltrate, scale-crust, and melanophages.[5] It is proposed that increased ketone bodies pass from the circulating blood into tissues or remain near the blood vessels, inducing cytotoxic effects and perivascular inflammation leading to the lesions seen in PP.[5,10,11]

With the increasing popularity of ketogenic diets for various reasons including weight loss and control of certain seizures, we might see an increase in PP cases. PP is a self-limiting condition with good prognosis when the trigger is avoided or treated. However, in severe cases, treatment may be required during the inflammatory phase. Oral dapsone, minocycline, doxycycline, and tetracycline all were reported to be beneficial by limiting the local tissue inflammatory response and cytotoxic effects. Topical and systemic antihistamines as well as corticosteroids are ineffective and have not been shown to prevent the postinflammatory reticular pigmentation. Introducing carbohydrate and thereby reducing ketosis helped in remission in many case reports including the case with our patient. In diabetic ketoacidosis, lesions were treated with introduction of insulin.[6-9]

CONCLUSION

Prurigo pigmentosa is rare yet increasingly recognized cause for an inflammatory intensely pruritic rash lasting for 1 week and heal with hyperpigmentation that resolve after few weeks. Causes include any state of ketosis such as a strict ketogenic diet. Diagnosis is through history and clinical presentation of erythematous rash involving the trunk, limbs, and sparing the mucous membranes. Histopathology of early lesions shows superficial perivascular and interstitial infiltrate of neutrophils followed by lymphocytic infiltration and necrosis of numerous keratinocytes then scale-crust, and melanophages at late stages. Introduction of carbohydrate results in resolution of symptoms within 1 week without treatment. However, treatment may be required early in the disease with oral dapsone, minocycline, or doxycycline.

KEY MESSAGES

- Always ask about dietary modifications in patients presenting with a new rash.
- Prurigo pigmentosa once considered rare is getting more common with the increase in ketogenic diets worldwide for various reasons including weight loss and control of seizures and therefore should be kept in the differential diagnosis of persistent intensely itchy rash.

REFERENCES

1. Nagashima M. Prurigo Pigmentosa—Clinical Observation of Our 14 Cases. J Dermatol. 1978;5(2):61-7.
2. James W, Berger T, Elston D. Andrews' Diseases of the Skin: Clinical Dermatology, 10th edition. Philadelphia: Saunders; 2005.
3. MDedge. (2019). Prurigo Pigmentosa Induced by Ketosis: Resolution Through Dietary Modification. [online] Available from https://www.mdedge.com/dermatology/article/196684/pigmentation-disorders/prurigo-pigmentosa-induced-ketosis-resolution. [Last accessed October, 2020].
4. Michaels JD, Hoss E, DiCaudo DJ, Price H. Prurigo pigmentosa after a strict ketogenic diet. Pediatr Dermatol. 2015;32(2):248-51.
5. Kim JK, Chung WK, Chang SE, Ko JY, Lee JH, Won CH, et al. Prurigo pigmentosa: clinicopathological study and analysis of 50 cases in Korea. J Dermatol. 2012;39(11):891-7.
6. Böer A, Ackerman AB. Prurigo Pigmentosa (Nagashima Disease): Textbook and Atlas of a Distinctive Inflammatory Disease of the Skin. New York, NY: Ardor Scribendi Ltd.; 2004.
7. Teraki Y, Teraki E, Kawashima M, Nagashima M, Shiohara T. Ketosis is involved in the origin of prurigo pigmentosa. J Am Acad Dermatol. 1996;34(3):509-11.
8. Oh YJ, Lee MH. Prurigo pigmentosa: a clinicopathologic study of 16 cases. J Eur Acad Dermatol Venereol. 2011;26(9):1149-53.
9. Yokozeki M, Watanabe J, Hotsubo T, Matsumura T. Prurigo pigmentosa disappeared following improvement of diabetic ketosis by insulin. J Dermatol. 2003;30(3):257-8.
10. VanItallie TB, Nufert TH. Ketones: Metabolism's ugly duckling. Annu Rev Nutr. 2003;61:327-41.
11. Hartman M, Fuller B, Heaphy MR. Prurigo Pigmentosa Induced by Ketosis: Resolution Through Dietary Modification. Cutis. 2019;103(3):E10-3.

CASE 4

Chronic Suffering from Undiagnosed Generalized Itching, Papules, and Plaques: The Relief Impact of a Single Dermoscope Examination

Gabriel Peres, Vidal Haddad Jr, Roberta Fachini Jardim Criado, Walter Belda Junior, Paulo Ricardo Criado

CASE PRESENTATION

A 78-years-old Caucasian female patient was referred to our dermatology clinic due to a history of cutaneous pruriginous recurrent lesions during the last year. She noticed serious impairment of her sleep caused by severe itching on several parts of her body, except on face and scalp. During the last 6 months, she had many outpatient consultations, receiving many attempts of treatment such as oral hydroxyzine, loratadine, topic, and systemic corticosteroids, topic, and systemic antibiotics, with mild and temporary relief of itch.

Additionally, she denied fever, weight loss, nausea, contact with animals and chemical products, and physical injuries. Absent previous history of environmental and laboral exposures, neither remarkable vaccine panel, recent trips and risky sexual behavior.

Her past medical history was marked by poorly controlled diabetes mellitus and systemic arterial hypertension. She also had a cervix genital cancer, 3 years before, treated with surgery and inguinal lymphadenectomy, without chemo- or radiotherapy. She denied pruritus or similar cutaneous lesions on any family members.

On dermatological examination, patient presented several erythematous–violaceous papules, plaques, squamous lesions, some of them eroded, excoriated, and ulcerated on her trunk and arms, there were also burrows on palms and writs (**Fig. 1A**). Excoriated papules on mammary areola were seen on both breasts. There was bilateral cervical lymphadenopathy. No oral or genital lesions were present.

Dermoscopy examination with 10× magnifications (DermLite DL100, 3Gen) of palms and excoriated papules of the dorsum showed excoriations and crusts, fine vessels neoformation secondary to reparative process in excoriated and ulcerates lesions of dorsum, which also demonstrated brown structures displaying delta wings configuration at the end of burrows in epidermis, a typical "delta wing jet with contrail" sign (**Fig. 2**). We performed her first cutaneous biopsy (not performed on previous consultations) for conventional histopathology essay, showing an eczematous cutaneous reaction with tissue eosinophilia, without mite

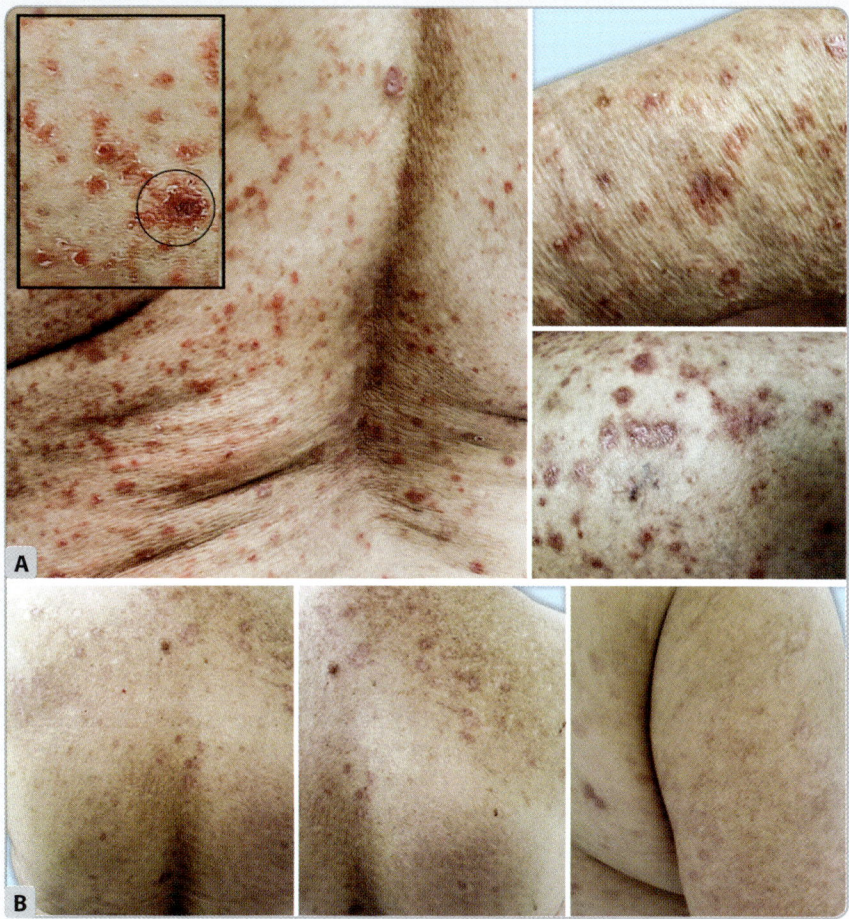

FIGS. 1A AND B: (A) Atypical clinical presentation of scabies *incognito*. A myriad of elementary lesions could be identified on this patient, turned a trouble the prompt diagnosis, achieved by dermoscopy clues. (B) After combined treatment, overall improvement, lasting only scaring and hyperchromic lesions.

structures. Direct immunofluorescence was performed to exclude nonbullous variant of bullous pemphigoid, considering the advanced age, uncommon chronic pruriginous lesions presentation, and immunoreactions negativity.

Correlating clinical, dermoscopic, and pathology findings for prurigo nodularis-like lesions, lichenoid papules, and nodules directed us to establish the diagnosis, of not only an atypical form of nodular scabies, but a scabies *incognito*, both subtypes of scabies surreptitious.

Treatment was performed with topical 5% permethrin cream applied over her entire body skin, except on face and scalp, over 8 hours per night, during 3 consecutive days and repeated after a week. Additionally, she received single dose of oral ivermectin 200 μg/kg, repeated after 2 weeks. The patient returned to our clinic, 20 days later, without complaints of pruritus, noticing normal sleep and showed only residual scars and hyperpigmented residual lesions on her skin (**Fig. 1B**).

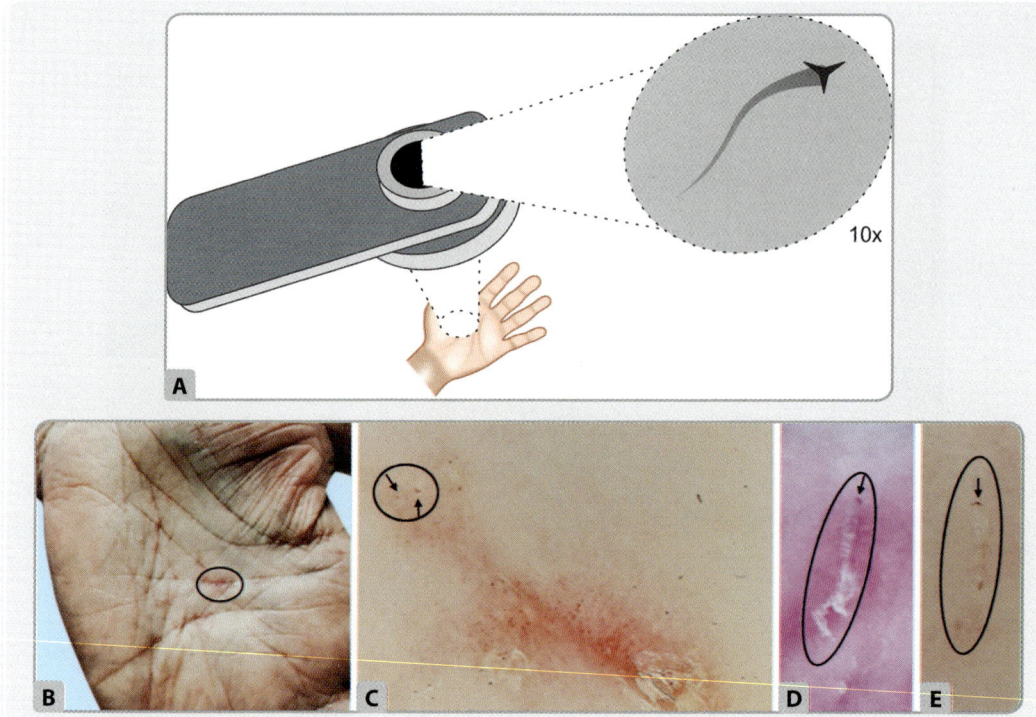

FIGS. 2A TO E: (A) Scheme of a 10× magnification dermoscopy focusing lesion with typical pattern of the "delta wing jet with contrail" sign. (B) Clinical examination of burrow on palm. (C to E) Dermoscopic pictures of female mites (arrow) and its burrows.

DISCUSSION

Sarcoptes scabiei variety *hominis* is a mite that causes scabies, an infestation in humans with over 300 million cases per year.[1] Scabies diagnosis is usually established following appropriate patient history and physical examination of specific skin lesions and their distribution (such as burrows often found in the finger space webs), and also the presence of classical clinical presentations characterized by generalized pruritus.[2] Unfortunately, in patients on treatment with potent topical corticosteroids or systemic steroids and/or with immunocompromising disorders, scabies can show atypical manifestations on the skin.[2] These unusual or atypical cutaneous findings of scabies are named as scabies surreptitious or scabies *incognito*.[1,2]

In this article, we describe the dermoscopy application as a useful method for complementary physical examination in the uncommon setting of patients with long-term severe pruritus caused by scabies *incognito*, whose skin lesions can mimic prurigo nodularis and lichenoid eruption.

The suspicion of scabies usually is made from a generalized pruritus claim, often more severe during the evening or night, in a patient with skin presenting burrows, which most often are localized to the interdigital web spaces, but may also be present in the axillae, on breasts, on the buttocks, on the elbows, on the flexor surfaces of the wrists.[1] Often, patients can demonstrate inflammatory papules, pustules, excoriations, and/or vesicles on affected areas.[1]

The main impact in scabies *incognito* is the severe itch and atypical lesions that causes remarkable suffering during a long time. It is not quite common to use a dermoscope to evaluate those clinical presentations.

Diagnosis of scabies is unequivocal with clinical characteristic lesions and findings of *Sarcoptes scabiei* variety *hominis* (gold standard), its excrement (*scybala*), or its eggs on microscopic examination skin scraping, and is thought to have a 100% specificity.[1,3]

Alternative diagnostic techniques include skin biopsy with findings of the entire mite (or parts) in the *stratum corneum*, burrow ink test, and polymerase chain reaction.[1] Noninvasive techniques are also possible, such as in vivo reflectance confocal microscopy, optical coherence tomography, and video dermoscopy, though expensive, time-consuming, and not always accessible for most dermatologists.[1]

Since sensitivity and negative predictive value of skin scraping are completely dependable of performer's expertise, especially in common scabies, when only few mites are scattered over the 1.9 m^2 of body surface, dermoscopy is a simple, fast, convenient, and cost-effective technique for screening large areas to find the mite's precise location.[3,4]

Originally, dermoscopy was employed to improve the detection of melanoma, now it has been used in a plethora of dermatologic conditions.[4] Digital dermoscopic photographs can be viewed and also magnified immediately on camera or computer screens.[4]

Argenziano et al.[3] first reported the dermoscopic "triangle sign," which represents the "head" portion of the mite, and "the delta wing jet with contrail" sign, corresponding to the head of the female mite and the trailing burrow, as seen on **Figure 2** scheme and pictures. Dermoscopy, at 10× magnification, is 91% sensitive [95% confidence interval (CI) 86–96%] and 86% specific (95% CI 80–92%) for scabies.[5]

At 20-40× magnifications, the typical appearance of the mite's head and two pairs of forelegs resemble the triangular shape of a hang-glider. Sometimes, the contour of the round body of the mite can also be identified.[6]

Chronic generalized pruritus leads to long-standing disease with severe impairment of sleep, quality of life, and interpersonal relationships. The true value of dermoscopy in such cases as scabies *incognito* is the ability of trained physicians magnify skin layers and achieve diagnosis 6× faster.[2]

Scabies surreptitious is a term that has recently been established to unify not only the numerous variants but also the atypical presentations of scabies, under distinct subtypes: Bullous, crusted, dermatitis herpetiformis-like, ecchymoses; hidden, *incognito*, Langerhans cell histiocytosis-like, nodular, pityriasis rosea-like, scalp, systemic lupus erythematosus-like, urticaria, urticaria pigmentosa-like.[7]

A recent study found that 45% of the patients presenting to the dermatology office with scabies had been misdiagnosed by another provider, resulting unnecessary costs for tests, treatment, and patients' long-standing suffering condition.[7,8] Increasing awareness of atypical scabies presentations can reduce the financial burden and the possible side effects of treatments due to an incorrect diagnosis.[7]

The 2017 European Guideline for the management of scabies recommends—(1) Permethrin 5% cream (repeat once after 7-14 days) or oral ivermectin 200 μg/kg (repeat after 7 days) or benzyl benzoate lotion 10–25% on days 1, 2, and repeat after 7 days; (2) Topical treatment should be applied to all skin regions at night and left in place for 8-12 hours; (3) Clothing, bedding, towels, etc., in machine washed, dry-cleaned, or sealed in plastic bag for 1 week, and (4) A follow-up visit 2 weeks after completion of treatment for a test of cure by microscopy examination.[9]

Recently, a Cochrane review[10] about permethrin and ivermectin treatment concluded that the efficacy of oral ivermectin (at a standard dose of 200 μg/kg) may lead to slightly lower rates of complete clearance after 1 week compared to permethrin 5% cream. Using the average clearance rate of 65% in the trials with permethrin, the illustrative clearance with ivermectin is 43% (RR 0.65, 95% CI 0.54–0.78; 613 participants,

6 studies; low-certainty evidence). The authors emphasized that they found that for the most part, there was no difference detected in the efficacy of permethrin compared to systemic or topical ivermectin.[10] Combination of topical treatment (e.g., permethrin) with oral ivermectin was not evaluated but can be an option for generalized lesions in the setting of scabies *incognito*.

Table 1 summarizes suspicion findings for scabies incognito in patients with long-standing

TABLE 1: Main suspicion findings for scabies incognito, workup, and treatment.

	Favors scabies	Against scabies
Main complaints	<ul><li>Severe pruritus</li><li>More intense during the night with sleep impairment</li></ul>	<ul><li>Pruritus associated with other clinical conditions (renal impairment, diabetes, neurologic and psychiatric conditions), or exposures (chemical, plants, physical agents, and insects)</li></ul>
Clinical examination	<ul><li>Erythematous papules (~2 mm)</li><li>Excoriations, crusts, and scales</li><li>Distribution on folds (mammary, axillae, inguinal, and buttocks) and hands</li></ul>	<ul><li>Bullae</li><li>Tumors and nodules</li><li>Photoexposed areas</li><li>Lesions with different evolution progression</li><li>Broad distribution</li><li>Sparing hands and folds</li></ul>
Dermoscopy	"Delta wing jet with contrail" sign	No specific signs
Main differential diagnosis for scabies incognito	Prurigo nodularis, lichenoid eruption, generalized contact dermatitis, pruritus hepaticus, renal pruritus, and nonbullous variant of bullous pemphigoid	
Unsuccessful therapies usually prescribed for similar conditions before scabies incognito diagnosis	<ul><li>Antihistamines (e.g., hydroxyzine, fexofenadine, and loratadine), topical and systemic corticosteroids (e.g., oral prednisone and clobetasol dipropionate 0.05% ointment)</li><li>*OBS*: Immunosuppressive drugs may relief but can be the cause of scabies incognito</li></ul>	
Workup (commonly available)	<ul><li>*Biopsy*: Conventional histopathology (hematoxylin and eosin stain) can show an eczematous cutaneous reaction with tissue eosinophilia, with or without mite structures</li><li>*Direct microscope examination*: Skin scrap with presence of the mite, its excrement (*scybala*), or eggs</li><li>*Laboratories*: Rule out systemic disease causing pruritus (minimum tests for renal and hepatic examinations, fasten glucose, and complete blood count)</li></ul>	
Scabies-specific treatments	Topical (applied to all skin regions, except face and the scalp, at night and left in place for 8–12 hours):<ul><li>*5% permethrin cream*: 3 days and repeated after 7–14 days</li><li>*Benzyl benzoate lotion 10–25%*: 2 days and repeated after 7 days</li></ul>Systemic:<ul><li>*Oral ivermectin 200 µg/kg*: Single dose and repeated after 7 days</li></ul>	

undiagnosed pruritus, also workup and treatment mainstay.

CONCLUSION

The long-standing course of scabies *incognito* has a severe impairment on quality-of-life of those patients. Dermoscopy-guided scraping and microscopic examination are easily accessible, permitting rapid approach for precise diagnosis and treatment of patients and their close contacts, thus decreasing the probability of infestation spread, thereby reinforcing the increasing importance of this technique in routine practice, in distinct clinical settings.

KEY MESSAGES

- Long-standing scabies *incognito* can cause severe impairment on quality-of-life.
- Dermoscopy-guided scraping and microscopic examination are useful for precise diagnosis and treatment.

REFERENCES

1. Werbel T, Hinds BR, Cohen PR. Scabies presenting as cutaneous nodules or malar erythema: reports of patients with scabies surrepticius masquerading as prurigo nodularis or systemic lupus erythematosus. Dermatol Online J. 2018;24:8.
2. Diab HM. Scabies incognito: diagnostic value of dermoscopy-guided microscopic examination. J Egypt Women Dermatol Soc. 2017;14:56-60.
3. Argenziano G, Fabbrocini G, Delfino M. Epiluminescence microscopy. A new approach to in vivo detection of Sarcoptes scabiei. Arch Dermatol. 1997;133:751-3.
4. Fox G. Diagnosis of scabies by dermoscopy. Case Reports. 2009:bcr0620080279.
5. Dupuy A, Dehen L, Bourrat E, Lacroix C, Benderdouche M, Dubertret L, et al. Accuracy of standard dermoscopy for diagnosing scabies. J Am Acad Dermatol. 2007;56:53-62.
6. Neynaber S, Wolff H. Diagnosis of scabies by dermoscopy. CMAJ. 2008;178:1540-1.
7. Stiff KM, Cohen PR. Scabies Surrepticius: Scabies Masquerading as Pityriasis Rosea. Cureus. 2017;9:e1961.
8. Anderson KL, Strowd LC. Epidemiology, Diagnosis, and Treatment of Scabies in a Dermatology Office. J Am Board Fam Med. 2017;30:78-84.
9. Salavastru CM, Chosidow O, Boffa MJ, Janier M, Tiplica GS. European guideline for the management of scabies. J Eur Acad Dermatol Venereol. 2017;31:1248-53.
10. Rosumeck S, Nast A, Dressler C. Ivermectin and permethrin for treating scabies. Cochrane Database Syst Rev. 2018;4:CD012994.

CASE 5

A Case of Pruritus with Symptomatic Dermographism Previously Treated as Eczema

*Ryo Saito, Hajime Shindo, Shunsuke Takahagi,
Akio Tanaka, Michihiro Hide*

CASE PRESENTATION

A 38-year-old man was referred to our department complaining of itchy small papules and scaling erythema on the scalp, chest, back, and legs. He had suffered from the symptoms for as long as about 20 years. They were refractory to treatment with topical corticosteroids and oral antihistamines (**Figs. 1A** and **B**). He had consulted several dermatologists and been diagnosed with pruritus with secondarily developed chronic eczema before visiting our department. He reported that the skin eruptions started to appear in his early teens as eczema on the arms, and repeated exacerbations and remissions. When he entered university, the eruptions began to be accompanied by severe systemic itching. He likened the symptoms to being stung by >100 insects, followed by rapid spreading and then disappearance of the wheals-and-flare in a few hours every evening. Confirming the appearance of wheal-like eruptions through a photo taken at home by the patient (**Fig. 1C**), we made a diagnosis of pruritus, chronic spontaneous urticaria, and/or prurigo. Consequently, we prescribed a double-dose of antihistamine, montelukast—a leukotriene receptor antagonist mainly aiming at urticaria, and topical corticosteroid for prurigo. The occurrence of wheals decreased to <10 per day within 2 days upon taking the medications. However, he still presented small papules and linear erythema. Light scratching of the skin revealed comorbidity of symptomatic dermographism (**Fig. 1D**).[1] Six months after the first visit, oral cyclosporine 125 mg (2 mg/kg) was added to manage the remaining urticaria. The development of papules and scaling erythema were further reduced in 6 weeks. He only suffered from occasional development of itchy small papules followed by consequential appearance of dermographism (**Figs. 2A** and **B**). He once stopped taking cyclosporine because of economic reasons and due to suspicions that it was ineffective, resulting in an exacerbation of the symptoms. He then restarted cyclosporine and then reachieved symptom control. A small itchy red papule which transiently developed on his buttock was biopsied (**Fig. 2A**). It showed normal epidermis and slight interstitial dermal edema with moderate superficial perivascular and interstitial infiltrate of eosinophils, neutrophils, and lymphocytes, being consistent with urticaria (**Fig. 2C**).

CASE 5 A Case of Pruritus with Symptomatic Dermographism Previously Treated as Eczema

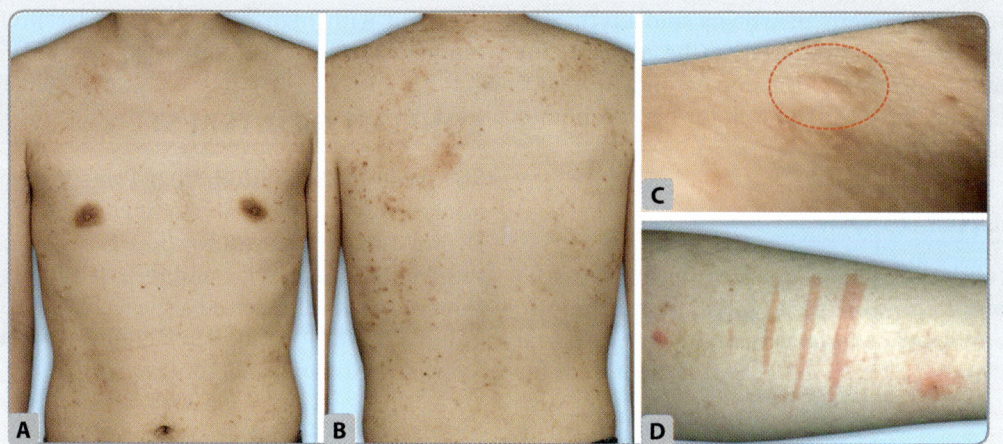

FIGS. 1A TO D: Itchy small papules and scaling erythema scattered on the chest and back (A and B). Wheals with strong itching developed on the leg (C). The linear erythema and wheals induced by scratch with FricTest®1(D).

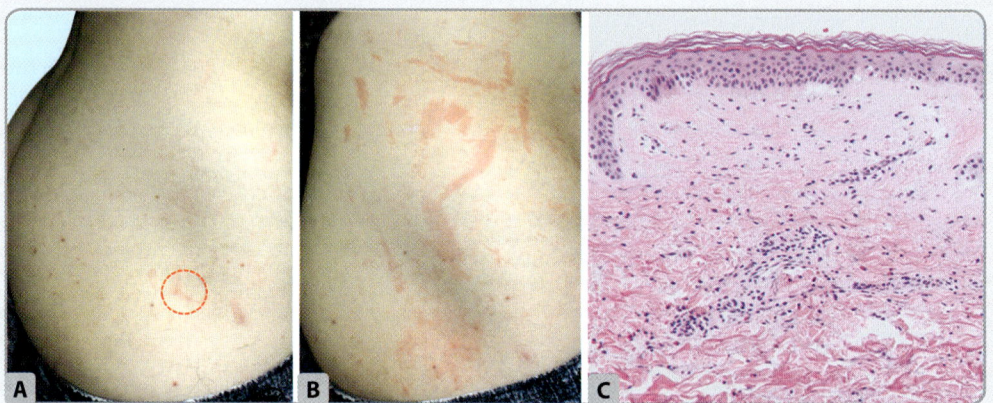

FIGS. 2A TO C: An itchy small wheal with a stinging sensation on his right buttock (A) turned into a wide erythematous wheal together with the appearance of many linear erythematous eruptions in as fast as 24 minutes (B). Slight interstitial dermal edema with superficial perivascular and interstitial infiltrate of eosinophils, neutrophils, and lymphocytes were observed by biopsy of the initial wheal lesion (C).

DISCUSSION

Here, we show a case presenting with itchy wheals, erythema, and secondarily developed papules, and scaling erythema. The skin eruption was atypical as either chronic spontaneous urticaria or chronic prurigo.[2,3] The biopsy of a skin lesion revealed histopathology consistent with urticaria, but not epidermal hyperplasia or hyperkeratosis to be observed in eczema and prurigo.[4] Since his atypical symptoms made it difficult to diagnose, for a long time, pruritus and chronic eczema had not been previously suspected. Topical corticosteroids were not effective for his symptoms, whereas oral double-dose antihistamines and montelukast partially improved them. The addition of oral cyclosporine further reduced the development of wheals and erythema. Cyclosporine is reported to be efficient for both of dermographism and chronic prurigo[5,6] and may have worked well for his compound disease state.

CONCLUSION

We diagnosed a patient with pruritus complicated with atypical symptomatic dermographism, which was refractory to topical steroids, but responded well to treatment for urticaria with high doses of antihistamine, montelukast, and cyclosporine.

CONFLICT OF INTEREST

MH received honorarium from Taiho Pharma, Mitsubishi-Tanabe, Teikoku-Seiyaku, Kaken, Kyowa Hakko Kirin, MSD, and Novartis. ST received a speaker's fee and research funding from Novartis. AT received a speaker's fee from Taiho Pharma, Mitsubishi-Tanabe Pharma, Kyowa Hakko Kirin, and Torii Pharm.

KEY MESSAGE

- Since symptoms can be atypical in compound disease states, it is important to distinguish each type of skin eruption.

REFERENCES

1. Schoepke N, Abajian M, Church MK, Magerl M. Validation of a simplified provocation instrument for diagnosis and threshold testing of symptomatic dermographism. Clin Exp Dermatol. 2015;40:399-403.
2. Hide M, Takahagi S. Urticaria and Angioedema in Fitzpatrick's dermatology, 9th edition. New York: McGraw-Hill Education; 2019. pp. 684-709.
3. Ständer HF, Elmariah S, Zeidler C, Spellman M, Ständer S. Diagnostic and treatment algorithm for chronic nodular prurigo. J Am Acad Dermatol. 2020;82:460-8.
4. Elder DE, Elenitsas R, Johnson BL, Murphy GF. Lever's Histopathology of the Skin, 9th edition. Philadelphia: Lippincott Williams and Wilkins; 2005. pp. 182-3; 245-6.
5. Toda S, Takahagi S, Mihara S, Hide M. Six cases of antihistamine-resistant dermographic urticaria treated with oral ciclosporin. Allergol Int. 2011;60: 547-50.
6. Wiznia LE, Callahan SW, Cohen DE, Orlow SJ. Rapid improvement of prurigo nodularis with cyclosporine treatment. J Am Acad Dermatol. 2018;78: 1209-11.

CASE 6

Immediate and Long-lasting Resolution of Pruritus and Skin Lesions by Targeting the IL-5 Receptor

*Guillet Carole, Steinmann Simona, Rosset Nina, Kolm Isabel,
Schmid-Grendelmeier Peter*

CASE PRESENTATION

A 12-year-old girl was referred to our dermatology clinic due to intensely pruritic, papulopustular dermatosis, which had been present for several years and had been continuously aggravating. The patient was otherwise healthy and physical examination showed no abnormal findings except skin changes (disseminated, excoriated erythematous papules, and pustules).

DIAGNOSTIC WORKUP

Skin biopsy specimen showed discrete pruritic changes of the epidermis and a marked dermal periadnexal and perivascular inflammatory infiltrate with the admixture of numerous eosinophilic granulocytes suggestive of eosinophilic perifolliculitis (**Fig. 1**), which might also be a special variant of atopic dermatitis.

Cytokine profiling of biopsy specimen showed elevation of interleukin (IL)-5 in skin. Laboratory testing showed significant blood eosinophilia [21.5%, normal range (NR) 0.0–7.0%; 3.3 G/L, NR 0.0–0.6) as well as elevated total serum immunoglobulin E (IgE) (maximum 1,978 kU/L, UNL 100 kU/L), soluble IL-5 (maximum 8.3 pg/mL, UNL 1 pg/mL), and eosinophilic cationic protein (ECP) [maximum 189 µg/mL (UNL 13.3 µg/mL)]. Elevation of eosinophil levels could be detected over a course of >6 months. There were no signs of hematologic malignancy, primary immunodeficiency, or secondary hypereosinophilia, excluded by extensive additional investigations including bone marrow aspiration. Organ involvement (e.g., cardial) was ruled out. Consequently, diagnosis of primary juvenile eosinophilic folliculitis was made.

TREATMENT

Treatment with topical and oral corticosteroids as well as indomethacin was initiated. Symptom control was unsatisfying over a course of several months and relapses after steroid tapering occurred very quickly. Due to markedly elevated eosinophilia in biopsy specimen and in blood and high levels of

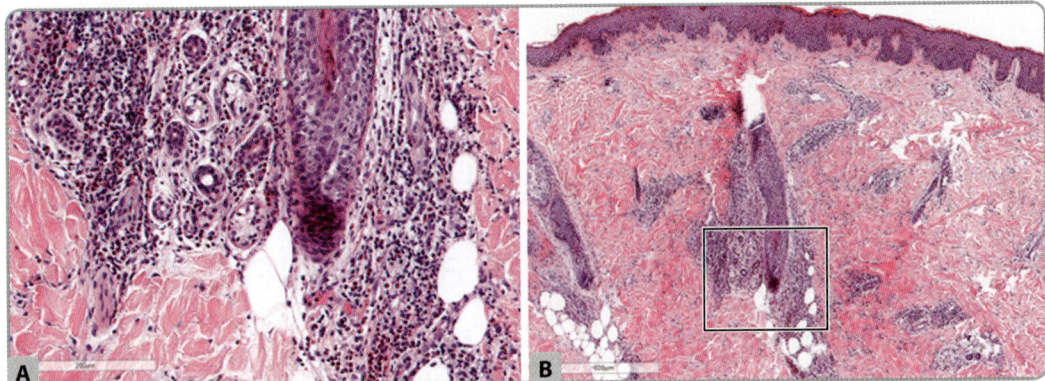

FIGS. 1A AND B: Biopsy of left shoulder; HE stain; showing a dense perifollicular and perivascular inflammatory infiltrate in the superficial and deep dermis. Close-up image shows the presence of multiple eosinophilic granulocytes in the infiltrate.

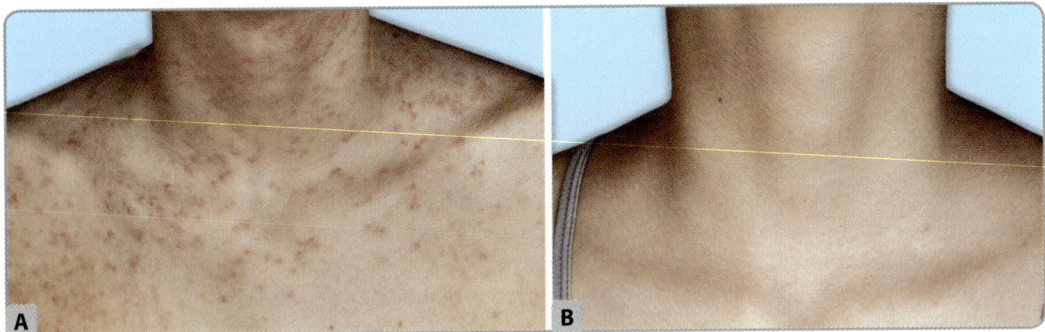

FIGS. 2A AND B: Neck before (left) and 4 weeks after (right) treatment with benralizumab.

interleukin-5 in both biopsy specimen and in serum, a single dose of benralizumab (=30 mg, subcutaneously) was administered. Pruritus resolved within 2 days. Skin changes and blood eosinophil count returned to normal within 4 weeks. Skin changes before benralizumab and 4 weeks after the first injection are shown in **Figures 2** to **4**.

The patient remained symptom-free for almost 6 months. Due to recurrence of pruritus and skin changes as of week 26 after the first injection, another dose of benralizumab was administered at week 30. Again, the itch and skin lesions improved within days and also the laboratory findings reflected this repeated response. Evolution of serum eosinophilia and serum ECP before and during treatment with benralizumab is summarized in **Table 1**.

DISCUSSION

Eosinophilic folliculitis is a chronic, noninfectious pruritic dermatosis of unknown etiology. It was first described by Ise and Ofuji in 1965.[1] It is characterized by sterile papulopustules predominantly found on face, neck, and chest.[2] Histologically, an eosinophilic infiltrate predominantly around the sebaceous glands can be found with occasional formation of eosinophil microabscesses.[3] Apart from the classic form of eosinophilic folliculitis affecting otherwise healthy and nonimmunocompromised individuals described by Ofuji in 1960, three additional variants of this disorder have been described:[4] (1) An infantile form with papulopustular lesions present predominantly on scalp, head, neck, and trunk,

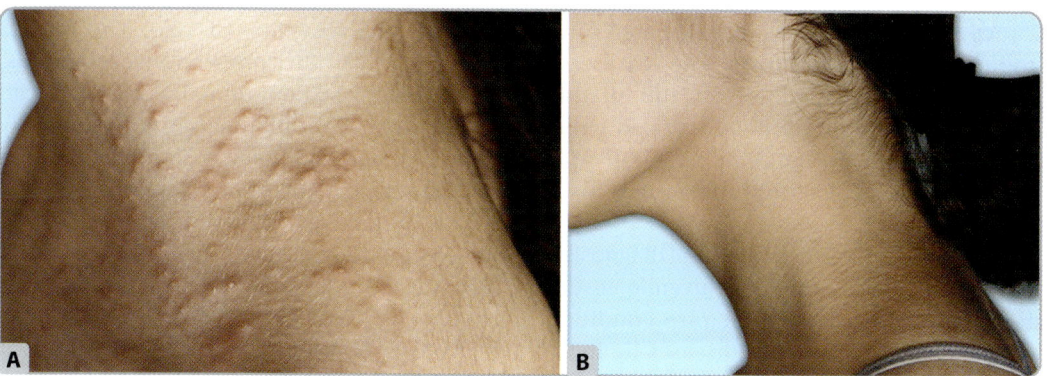

FIGS. 3A AND B: Left neck before (left) and 4 weeks after (right) treatment with benralizumab.

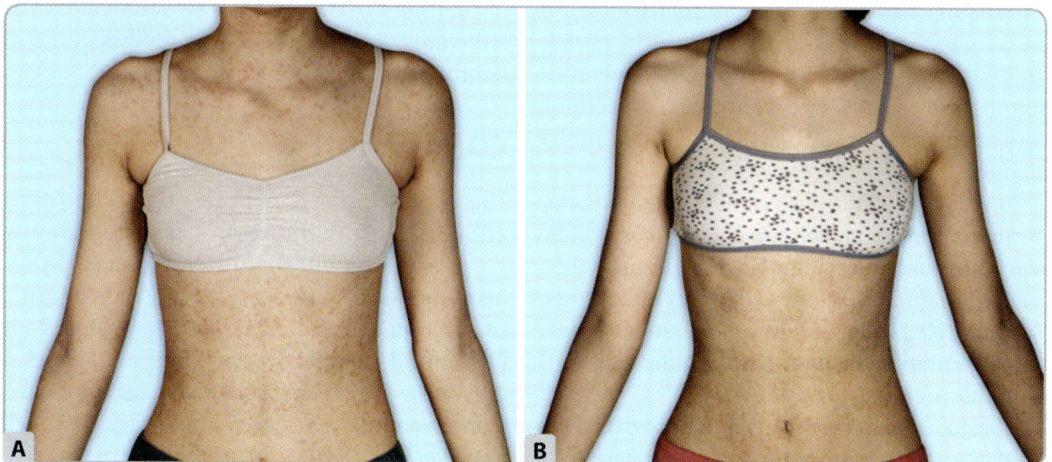

FIGS. 4A AND B: Trunk before (left) and four weeks after (right) treatment with benralizumab.

TABLE 1:	Eosinophilia and eosinophil cationic protein (ECP) before and during treatment with benralizumab.			
	Before TX with benralizumab	Week 4 after 1st benralizumab	Week 30 after benralizumab	4 weeks after 2nd benralizumab
Eosinophils in peripheral blood (NL: 0.0–0.6 g/L)	1.29 g/L (18%)	0.0 g/L	1.14 g/L	0.0 g/L
ECP (NL: <13.3 ug/L)	189 ug/L	11.11 ug/L	122.0 ug/L	9.6 ug/L

(NL: normal limits; TX: treatment)

(2) An immunosuppression-associated form, and (3) Drug-induced form. The features of our case were compatible with the infantile form of eosinophilic folliculitis, also called primary juvenile eosinophilic folliculitis. The pathogenesis of eosinophilic folliculitis is unknown.

In the wide range of differential diagnosis of eosinophilic dermatoses, the juvenile eosinophilic folliculitis is a rather rare condition. The majority of these skin diseases lie in the allergy-related group, including urticaria, allergic drug eruption, and atopic dermatitis. Another group of differential diagnosis are the eosinophilic dermatoses caused by parasitic infestations and arthropod bites such as scabies or larva migrans.[5] Besides these, skin-blistering diseases such as bullous pemphigoid and other autoimmune skin disorders as well as infectious and neoplastic diseases can lead to eosinophilia in the skin.[6]

Usually, juvenile eosinophilic folliculitis can be managed easily with topical corticosteroids. Various other treatments have been proposed including systemic steroids, topical tacrolimus, systemic dapsone, sulfonamides, macrolides, tetracyclines, cyclosporine, retinoids, and systemic and topical antifungals.[7]

Since in our patient, topical steroids were not sufficient and treatment with systemic steroids effective but not a considerable option in the long term, benralizumab was administered.

Benralizumab is a monoclonal antibody directed against the alpha-chain of the interleukin-5 receptor (CD125). The IL-5Rα chain is exclusively expressed by eosinophils, some basophils, and murine B1 cells, or B-cell precursors.[8] Benralizumab thus efficiently depletes blood and tissue eosinophils through antibody-dependent cell-mediated cytotoxicity. Benralizumab was approved by the US Food and Drug Administration (FDA) in November 2017, for the treatment of severe eosinophilic asthma.

Kuang Fl et al. have recently shown benralizumab to be highly effective in hyper-eosinophilic syndromes.[9] Use of mepolizumab, a monoclonal antibody against interleukin-5, has been shown to be highly effective in eosinophilic dermatoses.[10] However, in hypereosinophilic folliculitis, there have been no reports of use of benralizumab as a possible treatment.

CONCLUSION

The purpose of the present case report is to draw attention to the impressive fast therapeutic response of benralizumab and the long-lasting effect of almost 6 months considering the fact that benralizumab is administered for eosinophil-rich asthma needs every 8 weeks. Obviously, no reliable conclusion can be drawn from our experience in a single case. We feel, however, that in view of the rapid and impressive therapeutic response observed in our patient, it might be worthwhile to consider benralizumab administration in cases of therapy refractory eosinophilic folliculitis.

KEY MESSAGES

- Treatment of juvenile eosinophilic folliculitis with benralizumab has been shown to be highly effective in this patient.
- Benralizumab is a humanized monoclonal antibody targeted against the interleukin-5 receptor.
- Targeting the IL-5 and its receptor in eosinophilic dermatoses is a promising treatment with fast and long-lasting efficacy and further studies will be needed.

REFERENCES

1. Ise S, Ofuji S. Subcorneal pustular dermatosis. A follicular variant? Arch Dermatol. 1965;92:169-71.
2. Ofuji S, Ogino A, Horio T, Oseko T, Uehara M. Eosinophilic pustular folliculitis. Acta Derm Venereol. 1970;50:195-203.
3. Hernandez-Martin A, Nuno-Gonzalez A, Colmenero I, Torrelo A. Eosinophilic pustular folliculitis of infancy: a series of 15 cases and review of the literature. J Am Acad Dermatol. 2013;68:150-5.
4. Nervi SJ, Schwartz RA, Dmochowski M. Eosinophilic pustular folliculitis: A 40 year retrospect. J Am Acad Dermatol. 2006;55(2):285-9.
5. Long H, Zhang G, Wang L, Lu Q. Eosinophilic Skin Diseases: A Comprehensive Review. Clin Rev Allergy Immunol. 2016;50:189-213.
6. de Graauw E, Beltraminelli H, Simon HU, Simon D. Eosinophilia in Dermatologic Disorders. Immunol Allerg Clin N Am. 2015;35:545-60.
7. Nomura T, Katoh M, Yamamoto Y, Miyachi Y, Kabashima K. Eosinophilic pustular folliculitis: A published work-based comprehensive analysis of therapeutic responsiveness. J Dermatol. 2016;43:919-27.
8. Geijsen N, Koenderman L, Coffer PJ. Specificity in cytokine signal transduction: lessons learned from the IL-3/IL-5/GM-CSF receptor family. Cytokine Growth Factor Rev. 2001;12:19-25.
9. Kuang FL, Legrand F, Makiya M, Ware J, Wetzler L, Brown T, et al. Benralizumab for PDGFRA-Negative Hypereosinophilic Syndrome. N Engl J Med. 2019;380:1336-46.
10. Plotz SG, Simon HU, Darsow U, Simon D, Vassina E, Yousefi S, et al. Use of an anti-interleukin-5 antibody in the hypereosinophilic syndrome with eosinophilic dermatitis. N Engl J Med. 2003;349:2334-9.

CASE 7

An Unexpected Cause of Symptomatic Dermographism: Scabies

Esra Saraç, Emek Kocatürk

CASE PRESENTATION

A 30-year-old female patient presented with a complaint of swelling of her skin since 6 weeks. These swellings have been appearing exclusively after itching with a burning sensation and disappearing spontaneously in 1 hour. She had difficulty in sleeping because of the severe itching at night. Her medical history was not significant and she had no systemic disease. She had been treated with systemic antihistamines and topical emollients without any response.

SKIN EXAMINATION

Physical examination revealed linear urticarial plaques and excoriations on the extensor surfaces of the upper extremities. Dermographism was positive after rubbing a wooden tongue depressor to normal skin (**Fig. 1**; **Table 1**).

There were erythematous papules on the antecubital and axillary folds, the waist, and on the areolae, and brown irregular tracks in the palms and at the finger webs that were not mentioned by the patient, but were noticed during the dermatological examination (**Fig. 2**).

Further questioning of the patient on details about pruritus revealed that her spouse have been itching for the last 2 months too.

INVESTIGATIONS

Laboratory tests including complete blood count, basic biochemical tests, serum immunoglobulin E (IgE) level, and C-reactive protein were in normal ranges (**Table 2**).

Histopathological examination was not required as clinical and dermoscopic examination revealed light brown serpiginous burrow ending with a mite (**Fig. 3**).

DIAGNOSIS

Diagnosis of scabies and dermographism was made based on:
- *Clinical clues:*
  - Erythematous papules in the antecubital and axillary folds, waist, and areola.

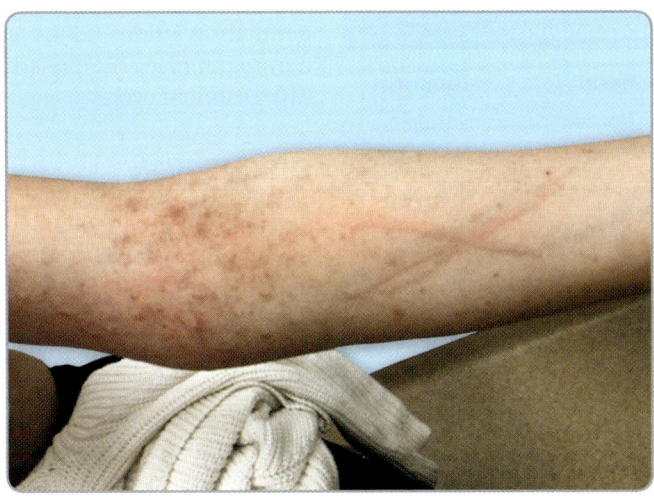

FIG. 1: Dermographism positive on volar surface of forearm along with the erythematous papules in the antecubital region.

TABLE 1: Physical examination.	
Test	Result
Dermographism	+
Involvement of antecubital and axillary folds, waist, and areola	+
Brown irregular tracks "burrows" in the palms and at the finger-webs	+
Dermoscopic findings	Burrow and mite at the end

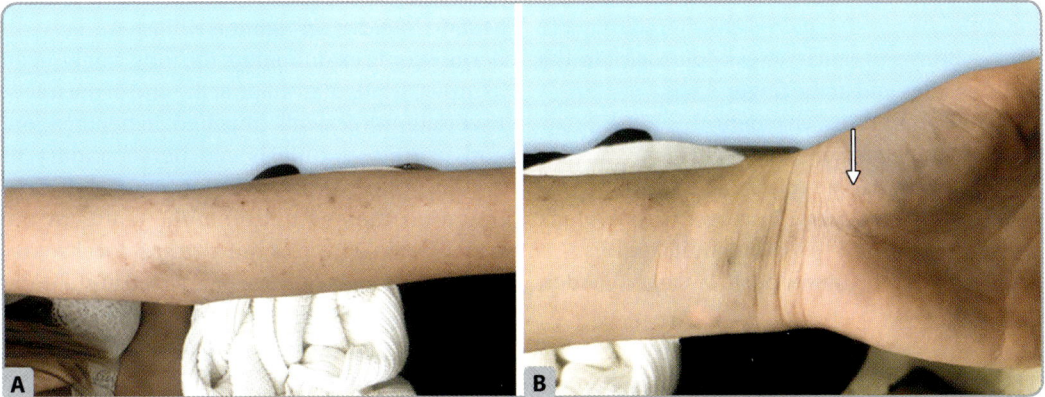

FIGS. 2A AND B: Erythematous papules on arms and brown irregular tracks in the palms (shown by the arrow).

TABLE 2:	Laboratory findings.	
Test	Result	Comment
Full blood count	Normal	Normal
CRP	3	Normal
Total IgE	86	Normal

(CRP: C-reactive protein; IgE: immunoglobulin E)

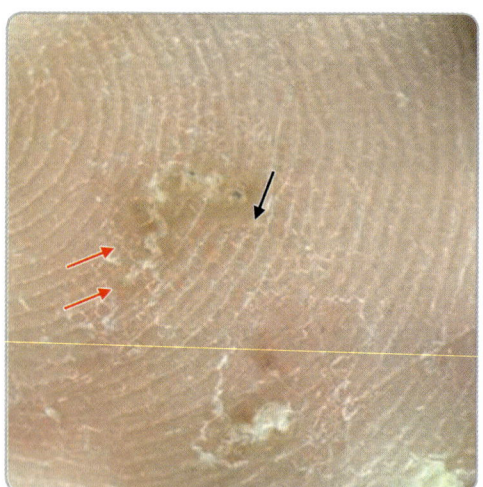

FIG. 3: Serpiginous burrow (red arrows) ending with mite (black arrow).
Courtesy: Ilkay Can.

- ○ Brown irregular tracks "burrows" in the palms and at the finger-webs
- ○ Symmetric involvement
- ○ Itching prominent at night
- ○ Itching in the spouse
- *Dermoscopic clues:* Burrows with a black head in the end "jetliner with its trail."

Dermographism was positive with a wooden tongue.

TREATMENT

The patient was treated topically with permethrin 5% lotion applied two courses with 1-week intervals. Itching decreased immediately after the first application of the permethrin lotion and the lesions as well as the dermographism disappeared completely after two treatment cycles.

DISCUSSION

Scabies is a cutaneous parasitosis caused by the microscopic mite, *Sarcoptes scabiei* variety *hominis*. This obligate ectoparasite completes its 10–14-day lifecycle in epidermis. Female mite spawns up to three eggs per day in stratum granulosum.[1] Symptoms and lesions are considered to be type-IV hypersensitivity reaction to the mite and its antigenic (egg, saliva, and feces) products.[2] The immune system with mast cells, complement system, eosinophils and T cells is involved in the complex pathomechanism of itch in scabies, which is the most prominent finding that exacerbates at night.[3] Pruritus generally starts within 6 weeks after first infestation, but this time interval may decrease to 24 hours in reinfestations.[4]

Erythematous papules and burrows are typical lesions concomitant to itching. Lesions are mostly located on interdigital spaces of hand, flexural surfaces of wrist and elbow, umbilicus, axillar and inguinal folds, thighs, waistline, genital area, and nipples. The burrows, where the mite travels through and lays its eggs, are pathognomonic for diagnosis. They present as short linear to serpiginous whitish tracks. With dermoscopic examination, the mite can be seen in brown triangular shape at the end of the tract.[5] Excoriations, eczema, impetigo, lichenification, and prurigo nodularis can be secondary to itching. Clinical presentation can be diverse based on the age and immune status of the patient. While head is not a typical localization for classical scabies, it can be affected in children, elderly, and immunocompromised individuals. Scabies can also present atypically with crust, bullae, and nodule formation. Distinguishing clinical features of scabies types and differential diagnosis are defined in **Table 3**.

Although symptomatic dermographism is not expected as a typical sign of scabies, it may be one of the clinical findings of the disease.[6,7]

TABLE 3: Types of scabies, prominent features, and differential diagnosis.

Type of scabies	Typical features	Differential diagnosis
Classical	• Lesions sparing scalp • Erythematous papules • Burrows	• Folliculitis • Atopic dermatitis • Contact dermatitis • Pediculosis corporis
Infantile	• Palmoplantar, scalp, and face involvement • Pustule, nodule formation	• Atopic dermatitis • Insect bite • Mastocytosis • Impetigo • Infantile acropustulosis • Langerhans cell histiocytosis
Crusted	• Hyperkeratotic crusted lesions • Mostly immunocompromised patient • High parasitic load • With or without pruritus • Erythroderma may exist	• Psoriasis • Palmoplantar keratoderma • Seborrheic dermatitis • Mycosis fungoides • Pityriasis rubra pilaris
Bullous	Bullae-vesicle formation	• Autoimmune bullous diseases • Insect bite
Nodular	• Genital area, axilla, and trunk • Persisting long	• Cutaneous lymphoma • Pseudolymphoma • Histiocytosis • Prurigo nodularis

The pathophysiology of the relationship between scabies and dermographism is unclear. Proteolytic enzymes that are secreted by the parasite might have led to direct stimulation and degranulation of the mast cells and occurrence of dermographism in this patient; this is supported by the disappearance of dermographism immediately after the clearance of mites from the skin.

Diagnosis of scabies is primarily based on dermatologic examination. Microscopy of skin scrapings and skin biopsy should be performed in the absence of pathognomonic clinical features. As well as dermoscopy, new generation noninvasive imaging techniques such as reflectance confocal microscopy, optical coherence tomography, and video dermoscopy can be used for the diagnosis.[8] The prevalence of scabies is reported between 0.2 and 71.4% depending on the different geographic regions.[9] Delay of the diagnosis may cause the mite to transmit to more people and result in outbreaks. In this context, it is important not to delay and treat the patient as early as possible. Epidemics in high-income countries frequently occur in institutional areas, homeless populations, and overcrowded groups who are living together after displacement. Children are excessively affected in low- and middle-income countries.[1]

The recommended first-line treatment options for scabies are permethrin 5% cream (on days 1, 8, and 15), benzyl benzoate 25% lotion (two consecutive days and reapplication after 1 week) or oral ivermectin (on days 1 and 8).

Topical treatment should be applied to dry and clean skin excluding the face and mucous membranes. Strictly ensuring personal and environmental hygiene is not only important for the success of the treatment but also for preventing reinfestations. All close contacts of the patient should be synchronously treated with topical scabicides regardless of having symptoms or not.

In crusted scabies, topical scabicides are applied daily for 1 week and then two times in a week until recovery, and also oral ivermectin is taken on days 1, 2, and 8. The length of the treatment might be extended for resistant cases.

In addition to these first-line treatments, malathion 0.5% lotion, ivermectin 1% lotion, sulfur 6–33% lotion, or synergized pyrethrin foam is also used as an alternative.[10]

CONCLUSION

Scabies must be excluded in every patient presenting with resistant pruritus regardless of the patient's socioeconomic level. The different clinical presentations of scabies should be kept in mind in order not to delay the diagnosis of this highly contagious infestation.

KEY MESSAGES

- Clinical presentation of scabies can differ in different patients.
- Scabies should be included in the differential diagnosis of all patients with resistant pruritus.

REFERENCES

1. Thomas C, Coates SJ, Engelman D, Chosidow O, Chang AY. Ectoparasites: Scabies. J Am Acad Dermatol. 2020;82:533-48.
2. Hengge UR, Currie BJ, Jäger G, Lupi O, Schwartz RA. Scabies: a ubiquitous neglected skin disease. Lancet Infect Dis. 2006;6:769-79.
3. Jannic A, Bernigaud C, Brenaut E, Chosidow O. Scabies Itch. Dermatol Clin. 2018;36:301-8.
4. Walton SF. The immunology of susceptibility and resistance to scabies. Parasite Immunol. 2010;32:532-40.
5. Cinnotti E, Perrot JL, Labeille B, Cambazard F. Diagnosis of scabies by high-magnification dermoscopy: the "delta-wing jet" appearance of *Sarcoptes scabiei*. Ann Dermatol Venereol. 2013;140:722-3.
6. Burkhart CN, Burkhart CG, Morrel DS. Infestations. In: Bolognia JL, Jorizzo JL, Schaffer JV (Eds). Dermatology, 3rd edition. China: Elsevier; 2012.
7. Taskapan O, Harmanyeri Y. Evaluation of patients with symptomatic dermographism. J Eur Acad Dermatol Venereol. 2006;20:58-62.
8. Micali G, Lacarrubba F, Verzi AE, Chosidow O, Schwartz RA. Scabies: Advances in Noninvasive Diagnosis. PLos Negl Trop Dis. 2016;10:e0004691.
9. Romani L, Steer AC, Whitfeld MJ, Kaldor JM. Prevalence of scabies and impetigo worldwide: a systematic review. Lancet Infect Dis. 2015;15(8):960-7.
10. Salavastru CM, Chosidow O, Boffa MJ, Janier M, Tiplica GS. European guideline for the management of scabies. J Eur Acad Dermatol Venereol. 2017;31:1248-53.

CASE 8

Intensive Pruritus, Excoriations and Inflammatory Papules Masking Dermatitis Herpetiformis

Maia Gotua, Elene Kakabadze

CASE PRESENTATION

We report a case of a 38-year-old woman with 13 years history of recurrent intensely pruritic eruption started after her first delivery. The eruption was characterized by intense itching and burning sensation in the erythematous papules, grouped vesicles, and tense blisters presented on elbows, buttocks, face, decollete area, and a back. The gastrointestinal symptoms were mildly presented. She has periodical exacerbations with intensive itching and skin manifestations—multiple excoriated papules, vesicles, erosions, and crusts mainly presented on her elbows, buttocks, back, and face.

Four years ago, after the second delivery, her symptoms exacerbated more. The symmetric intensive pruritic vesicular eruption on elbows, buttocks, face, decollete area, and back restarted. She has been diagnosed and treated as scabies, arthropod bites, atopic dermatitis, and contact dermatitis for many years (**Figs. 1A** to **E**). She presented to our clinic to exclude allergy. All allergy tests were negative.

Immunoglobulin A (IgA)-anti-transglutaminase 2 was 10 times more than the normal range (108 U/mL; normal range 7–10 U/mL). Besides, we concurrently measured total IgA levels. It was in the normal range. In patients with IgA deficiency, we perform IgG-based testing with deamidated gliadin peptide IgG. Jejunal biopsy, while the patient was on a gluten-containing diet, revealed villous atrophy characteristic for celiac disease; however, gastrointestinal symptoms were mildly presented. Skin biopsy in DH patients usually reveals granular IgA deposits. Skin lesions were very itchy and the patient was against doing the skin biopsy.

The skin lesions completely improved after a gluten-free diet (**Fig. 1F**).

118 SECTION 2 Interesting Cases: Pruritus

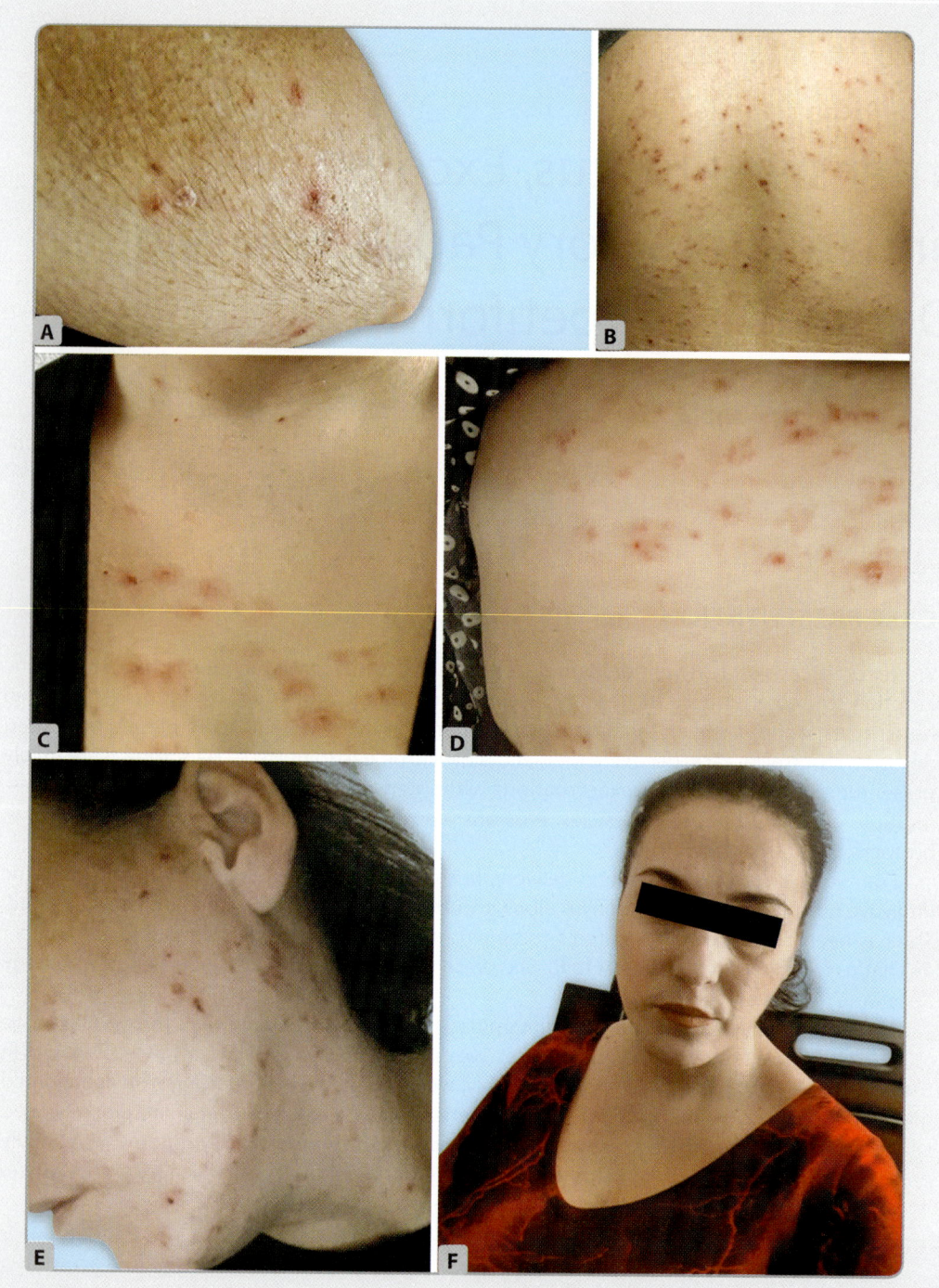

FIGS. 1A TO F: Skin lesions in the patient.

DISCUSSION

Dermatitis herpetiformis (DH) or Duhring–Brocq disease is a chronic, autoimmune blistering disease that appears as a cutaneous manifestation of gluten intolerance.[1] Celiac disease, also known as gluten-sensitive enteropathy, is an autoimmune, inflammatory disease of the small intestine caused by sensitivity to dietary gluten and related proteins in genetically predisposed individuals.[2,3] DH is a skin manifestation of celiac disease that classically presents as a symmetric pruritic vesicular eruption on extensor surfaces. The typical locations include elbows, upper forearms, knees, buttocks, and other parts of the body.[4] Facial and groin involvement has been reported rarely.[5,6]

Dermatitis herpetiformis, described as "celiac disease of the skin," is a cutaneous manifestation of gluten-sensitive enteropathy (celiac disease). Genetic predisposition and gluten-sensitivity are key factors in the pathogenesis of DH. Virtually all patients with DH carry the HLA DQ2 or HLA DQ8 haplotype. Antibodies against epidermal transglutaminase produced in association with an immune response to ingested gluten play a key role in the disease pathogenesis.[4,6-9] Affected patients typically develop intensely pruritic inflammatory papules and grouped vesicles (herpetiform) on the elbows, forearms, knees, buttocks, back, and scalp, which are common sites for lesion development.[4,8,9] The vast majority of patients with DH also have an associated gluten-sensitive enteropathy (celiac disease). In most of these patients, the enteropathy is minimally symptomatic or asymptomatic. Asymptomatic celiac disease was noted in 75–90% of patients with DH.[7-9] Our patient had mild symptoms of gluten-sensitive enteropathy. Patients with DH may have an increased risk for the development of other autoimmune diseases. Thyroid disease is the most common autoimmune disorder associated with DH. Patients with DH may also have an increased risk for lymphoma.[4,8,9]

Dermatitis herpetiformis is an uncommon autoimmune cutaneous disorder. It is frequently misdiagnosed as eczema, scabies, and another inflammatory skin disorder. Both skin conditions manifest as a highly itchy and bumpy rash that people often scratch. Intense pruritus is the predominant symptom; however, DH is a clinical chameleon and can cause excoriations, eczematous lesions, or minimal patterns of discrete erythema or digital purpura.[6,8,9] The clinical features of DH can resemble the clinical findings of other dermatologic disorders. Intensely pruritic conditions that present with excoriations and inflammatory papules, such as atopic dermatitis, scabies, and arthropod bites should be considered.[4,9]

Other subepidermal blistering diseases such as bullous pemphigoid, linear IgA bullous dermatosis, and bullous systemic lupus erythematosus are also included in the differential diagnosis. Blistering tends to be more prominent in these conditions than in DH. However, in the prodromal phase of bullous pemphigoid, blistering may be minimal or absent.[4,8,9]

The careful assessment of the patient history as well as the clinical, histopathologic, immunopathologic, and serologic findings usually successfully distinguishes DH from other disorders. The gold standard test for diagnosis of DH is direct immunofluorescence (DIF) of perilesional skin. DIF classically demonstrates granular deposits of IgA within the papillary dermis. Serologic studies that identify circulating IgA antibodies against tissue transglutaminase, epidermal transglutaminase, and endomysium are useful for confirming the diagnosis.[4,6,9] The diagnosis of celiac disease is established by the presence of increased intraepithelial lymphocytes with crypt hyperplasia (Marsh type 2) alone, or in conjunction with villous atrophy (Marsh type 3) on small bowel biopsy in a patient with positive celiac serology. However, villous atrophy can be patchy, and may also be present in a variety of other disorders that should be considered in the appropriate clinical settings. tTG-IgA serology may occasionally be positive but the small intestinal biopsy may not be normal or equivocal (Marsh 0 or 1, respectively). In patients with celiac disease and discordant serology and biopsy results, the intestinal biopsy should be re-reviewed by a pathologist familiar with celiac disease to look for subtle abnormalities of celiac disease. Besides, an alternate antibody test (EMA-IgA or DGP-IgA) should be performed. If serology and histology remain discordant, HLA-DQ2/DQ8 typing is needed to guide additional evaluation.[4,8,9]

Dermatitis herpetiformis usually responds well to treatment. Dapsone and a gluten-free diet are the primary interventions for the management of this disease. In our case, the only gluten-free diet was enough to control completely the symptoms of our patient with DH (**Fig. 1F**).

CONCLUSION

Dermatitis herpetiformis is a clinical chameleon characterized by intense itching and burning sensation in the erythematous papules, grouped vesicles, tense blisters, excoriations, eczematous lesions presented on elbows, forearms, knees, buttocks, back, scalp, face, and other parts of the body. Intensely pruritic conditions that present with excoriations and inflammatory papules, such as atopic dermatitis, scabies, and arthropod bites, should be considered for differential diagnosis. Other subepidermal blistering diseases should be considered as well.

KEY MESSAGES

- Extreme pruritus is a clinical hallmark of dermatitis herpetiformis.
- Due to the pruritus and intensive scratching, excoriations and erosions are often the most prominent clinical manifestations masquing dermatitis herpetiformis.

REFERENCES

1. Herrero-González JE. Clinical guidelines for the diagnosis and treatment of dermatitis herpetiformis. Actas Dermosifiliogr. 2010;101:820-6.
2. Mendes FBR, Hissa-Elian A, Abreu MAMM, Gonçalves VS. Review: dermatitis herpetiformis. An Bras Dermatol. 2013;88:594-9.
3. do Vale ECS, Dimatos OC, Porro AM, Santi CG. Consensus on the treatment of autoimmune bullous dermatoses: dermatitis herpetiformis and linear IgA bullous dermatosis - Brazilian Society of Dermatology. An Bras Dermatol. 2019;94(2 Suppl 1):48-55.
4. Hull C. (2020). Dermatitis herpetiformis. [online] Available from https://www.uptodate.com/contents/dermatitis-herpetiformis. [Last accessed October, 2020].
5. Cinats AK, Parsons LM, Haber RM. Facial Involvement in Dermatitis Herpetiformis: A Case Report and Review of the Literature. J Cutan Med Surg. 2019;23:35.
6. Pizzorno JE, Murray MT, Bey HJ. Dermatitis Herpetiformis in The Clinician's Handbook of Natural Medicine, 3rd edition. St. Louis, Missouri: Churchill Livingstone; 2016:245-8.
7. Samasca G, Baican A, Pirvan A, Miu N, Dejica D. Celiac Disease with Dermatitis Herpetiformis Case Report. J Biomol Res Ther. 2012;1(1):1-2.
8. Husby S, Murray JA, Katzka DA. AGA Clinical Practice Update on Diagnosis and Monitoring of Celiac Disease-Changing Utility of Serology and Histologic Measures: Expert Review. Gastroenterology. 2019;156:885-9.
9. Al-Toma A, Volta U, Auricchio R, Castillejo G, Sanders D, Cellier C, et al. European Society for the Study of Coeliac Disease (ESsCD) guideline for coeliac disease and other gluten-related disorders. United European Gastroenterol J. 2019;7(5):583-613.

CASE 9

Diagnosis and In Vivo Detection of *Sarcoptes Scabiei* by Dermoscopy

Sushrut Save, Kiran Godse

CASE PRESENTATION

A 21-year-old man presented with complaints of itchy red raised lesions over the web spaces of both hands since 2 months (**Fig. 1**). He also complained of similar lesions over the genitals associated with pruritus. He gave history of nocturnal exacerbation of itching. He had previously used multiple topical steroidal cream preparations and oral antihistamines with temporary relief. He gave history of similar complaints in his younger brother.

Cutaneous examination showed the presence of multiple erythematous to hyperpigmented papules and excoriations present in the web spaces of both hands. The genitals revealed the presence of erythematous papules over the scrotum and penis along with the presence of erythematous nodules over the glans.

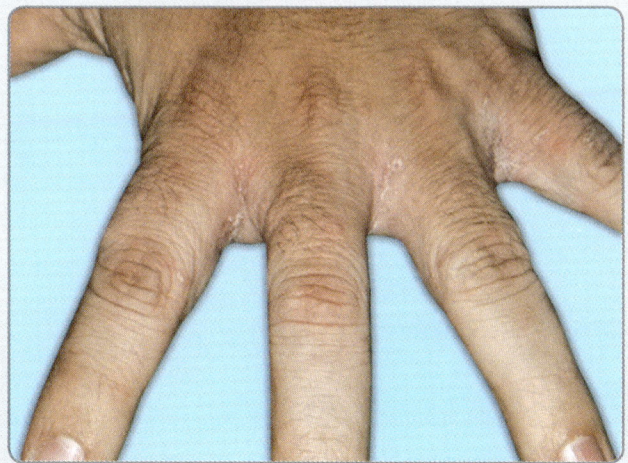

FIG. 1: Erythematous crusted papules and excoriations present in the web spaces of hand.

The dermoscopic examination of the hand lesions was done with Dermalite DL3N (10× magnification), which revealed the typical "triangular sign," which is basically a brown triangular structure at the end of a white, structureless wavy line (**Fig. 2**). The structureless whitish line is representative of the burrow.

A closer view of the triangular tip showed the presence of the scabietic mite present at the end of the translucent white line (**Fig. 3**). Hence, a diagnosis of scabies was confirmed.

The patient was first counseled regarding his personal hygiene as well as the hygiene of his immediate surroundings. He was advised a single dose of oral ivermectol 12 mg tablet to be repeated in the following week. He was also asked to apply topical permethrin 5% cream overnight along with a repeat application after 10 days. An oral antihistamine was also prescribed to counter his pruritus. Additionally, his family members were also advised to undergo therapy as a preventive measure. There was significant improvement in the symptoms at the end of 10 days.

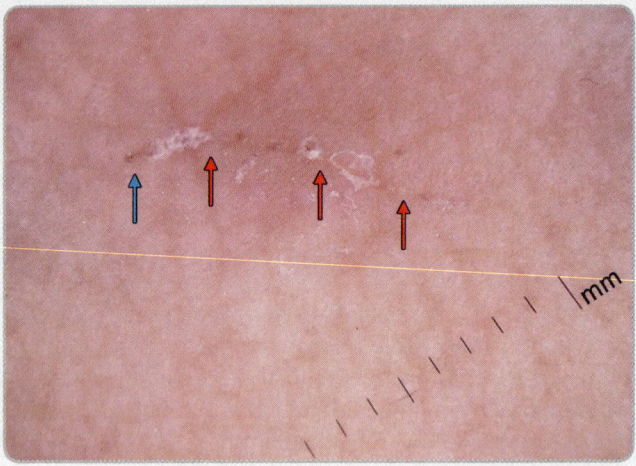

FIG. 2: Dermoscopic examination (10×) demonstrating the burrow as a wavy, whitish translucent line (red arrow), with a brown triangular tip (blue arrow).

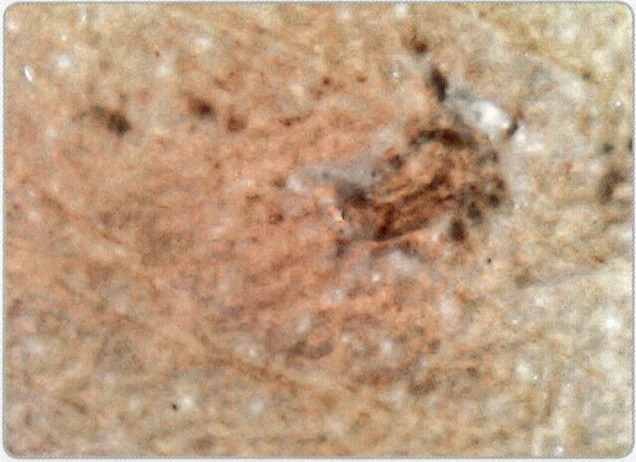

FIG. 3: The brown triangular tip under high magnification (20×) shows the presence of the mother mite.

DISCUSSION

Scabies is a contagious condition caused by the mite *Sarcoptes scabiei* variety *hominis*, and is known to affect people of all ages.[1,2] The diagnosis is usually quite straightforward owing to the typical presentation of lesions along with the history of nocturnal aggravation of itching and by microscopic examination of the burrow contents.[3] However, the microscopic examination is often time-consuming and cumbrous.[3] In such situations, dermoscopy may prove useful for a quick diagnosis with no down time, where other differential diagnosis such as atopic dermatitis may also be considered.[3] The typical dermoscopic features are the presence of burrows, which appear as wavy, white translucent lines with a brown triangular tip.[4] The burrows are essentially transepidermal tunnels, which are created due to the motion of the female mite.[5] The brown triangular tip at the end of the burrow represents the mite, and this appearance is also called the "triangle sign."[5,6]

The entire appearance of the brown tip along with the translucent white line has also been referred to as the "contrail" sign or the "delta glider" sign.[6] At times, the scabies eggs are also seen along the length of the burrows as tiny ovoid structures and some of these scabietic eggs may mature and demonstrate the minute heads of the maturing mite from within the egg, referred to as "minitriangle sign."[4,7]

CONCLUSION

Dermoscopy offers several advantages and benefits for the rapid and convenient diagnosis of scabies.[8] The patient compliance is also higher in case of dermoscopy-based diagnosis, in contrast to the existing diagnostic methods wherein skin scrapings or adhesive tape stripping are required which often tend to get cumbersome. It may also assist in better localization of the mite, which ensures higher diagnostic accuracy on detection by skin scraping.

KEY MESSAGE

- Dermoscopy has a high sensitivity, specificity, and positive–predictive value for the diagnosis of scabies and serves as an important instrument for diagnosis of suspected cases of scabies presenting with an atypical clinical picture and complaints of nonspecific pruritus all over the body.

REFERENCES

1. Burkhart CG, Burkhart CN, Burkhart KM. An epidemiologic and therapeutic reassessment of scabies. Cutis. 2000;65:233-40.
2. Hicks MI, Elston DM. Scabies. Dermatol Ther. 2009;22:279-92.
3. Malakar S. Dermoscopy Text and Atlas, 1st edition. New Delhi. Jaypee Brothers Medical Publishers (P) Ltd.; 2019. pp. 178-81.
4. Argenziano G, Fabbrocini G, Delfino M. Epiluminescence microscopy. A new approach to in vivo detection of *Sarcoptes scabiei*. Arch Dermatol. 1997;133:751-3.
5. Fox G. Diagnosis of scabies by dermoscopy. BMJ Case Rep. 2009;10:1136.
6. Prins C, Stucki L, French L, Saurat JH, Braun RP. Dermoscopy for the in vivo detection of *Sarcoptes scabiei*. Dermatology. 2004;208:241-3.
7. Dupuy A, Dehen L, Bourrat E, Lacroix C, Benderdouche M, Dubertret L, et al. Accuracy of standard dermoscopy for diagnosing scabies. J Am Acad Dermatol. 2007;56:53-62.
8. Walter B, Heukelbach J, Fengler G, Worth C, Hengge U, Feldmeier H. Comparison of dermoscopy, skin scraping, and the adhesive tape test for the diagnosis of scabies in a resource-poor setting. Arch Dermatol. 2011;147:468-73.

CASE 10

Prurigo Nodularis Treated Successfully with Dupilumab: Case Report and Review of the Literature

Jennifer Astrup Sørensen, Jesper Grønlund Holm, Simon Francis Thomsen

CASE PRESENTATION

A 52-year-old white man presented to our department in May 2015, with a 1-year history of itchy rash. He was diagnosed with prurigo nodularis (PN) in June 2015, and had a history of asthma since early childhood and rhinitis, but not atopic dermatitis (AD). Between 2015 and 2020, he was treated insufficiently with numerous medications including topical corticosteroids, oral antihistamines, ultraviolet light B (UVB), psoralen + ultraviolet light A (PUVA), prednisolone, azathioprine, gabapentin, acitretin, and thalidomide. Azathioprine caused nausea and heartburn and thalidomide was associated with disturbances in sensory nerve electrophysiology but not clinical neuropathy.

In June 2020, the patient had a Dermatology Life Quality Index (DLQI) score of 14 (out of 30), corresponding to severe impact on the quality of life, and an overall disease bother score of 7 out of 10 and an overall itch score of 10 out of 10 on a visual analogue scale (VAS). Treatment with dupilumab was initiated at an initial dose of 600 mg and then 300 mg every other week. At follow-up after 3 months, the patient reported clearance of symptoms, marked improvement in skin lesions (**Fig. 1**), and significant improvement in symptom scores with a DLQI score of 0, an overall disease bother score VAS of 1, and an itch VAS score of 0. He reported no side effects of the treatment (**Table 1**).

CASE 10 Prurigo Nodularis Treated Successfully with Dupilumab: Case Report and Review...

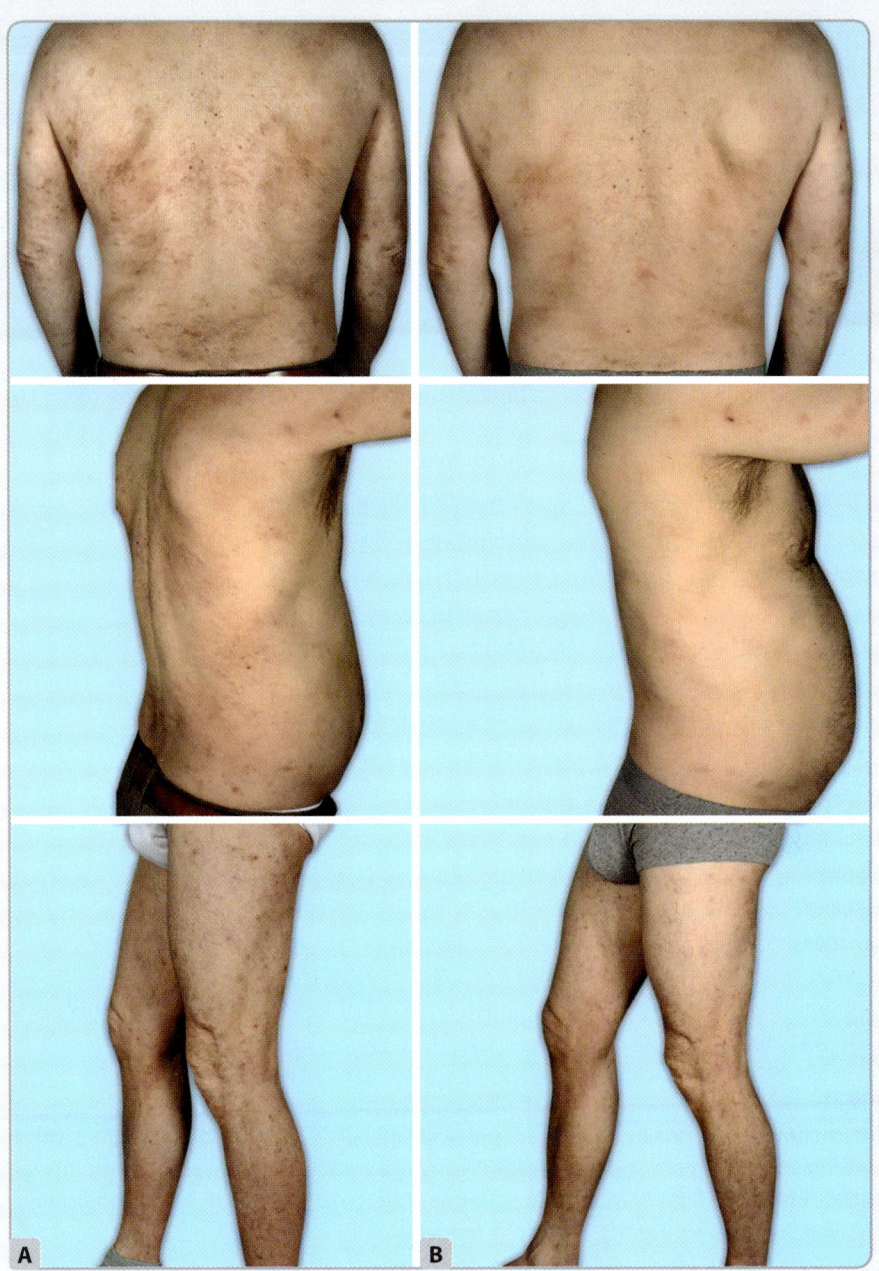

FIGS. 1A AND B: Patient at baseline (left) and at 3 months' follow-up (right).

TABLE 1:	Patient characteristics.
Sex	Male
Age (years)	52
Atopic dermatitis	No
Asthma	Yes
Allergic rhinoconjunctivitis	Yes
Sensitizations (RAST)	Birch, grass, horse, cat, alternaria
Serum total IgE	273 IU/L
Duration of PN (years)	6
Previous treatments	Topical corticosteroids, oral antihistamines, UVB, PUVA, prednisolone, azathioprine, gabapentin, acitretin, and thalidomide
Dupilumab treatment	Initial dose: 600 mg Maintenance dose: 300 mg every 2 weeks
Treatment duration	3 months (ongoing)
Follow-up	Complete effect. No itch
Overall effect	↑↑↑
PGA at follow-up	1
VAS	
• Overall disease bother score	
○ Baseline	7
○ 3 months	1
• Itch score	
○ Baseline	10
○ 3 months	0
DLQI	
Baseline	14
3 months	0
Side effects	None
[DLQI: Dermatology Life Quality Index; PGA; physician global assessment (scale of 1 to 5 with a higher score indicating more severe disease); PN: prurigo nodularis; PUVA: psoralen + ultraviolet light A; UVB: ultraviolet light B; VAS: visual analogue scale, 0–10, with a higher score indicating severe impact, Overall effect: → no effect, ↑ mild, ↑↑ moderate, ↑↑↑ complete]	

LITERATURE REVIEW

A systematic literature search in PubMed using the terms "prurigo nodularis" and "dupilumab" identified 14 publications in English (3 clinical cohorts, 6 case series, and 5 case reports) with a total of 59 patients exploring treatment with dupilumab for PN (**Table 2**). Overall, the treatment was well tolerated with clearance or almost clearance of symptoms in most of the patients.

DISCUSSION

Prurigo nodularis is an inflammatory skin disease characterized by nodule formation and chronic pruritus. Patients with PN suffer from poor quality of life due to the long-lasting, intense pruritus.[1] There are only limited options with regard to treatment and usually these have insufficient effect and/or severe side effects. Dupilumab is a fully human monoclonal antibody targeting the interleukin (IL)-4R approved for moderate/severe AD. Numerous studies have reported itch reduction in patients with AD, treated with dupilumab,[2] and recently an increasing number of studies have reported an effect of dupilumab in patients with PN.

We present a case of a 52-year-old male with long-standing PN, insufficiently controlled on numerous treatments. Following a flare-up of symptoms in the spring of 2020 he was started on dupilumab, with complete response already after 3 months and no reported side effects. A growing body of literature (a total of 60 patients published to date including our present case) suggests dupilumab as a promising treatment option in PN, with an increasing number of studies reporting good or excellent effect of treatment with few or no side effects.[3,4] Less data is available on the long-term effects of dupilumab for PN, and potential approval for clinical use awaits Phase III trials currently being conducted (EudraCT Number: 2019-003774-41/ 2019-003801-90).

CONCLUSION

Dupilumab appears to be a safe and effective treatment alternative for patients with PN often suffering from long-standing uncontrolled symptoms and severe impact on quality of life.

TABLE 2: Published literature on prurigo nodularis treated with dupilumab.

Study	Patients (females)	Age (years)	Atopic disease	Treatment dose	Efficacy	Adverse effects
Wieser et al.[5]	3 (2)	65.3	No	NA	3×↑	None
Romano[6]	1 (1)	61	No	600 mg induction, 300 mg every 2 weeks	↑↑↑	None
Criado et al.[7]	1 (0)	87	Yes	600 mg induction, 300 mg every 2 weeks	↑↑↑	None
Kovacs et al.[8]	1 (1)	80	Yes	600 mg induction, 300 mg every 2 weeks	↑↑↑	None
Holm et al.[9]	3 (3)	49	No	600 mg induction, 300 mg every 2 weeks	2×↑↑↑ 1×↑↑↑	None
Giura et al.[10]	1 (1)	85	No	600 mg induction, 300 mg every 2 weeks	↑↑↑	None

Continued

Continued

Study	Patients (females)	Age (years)	Atopic disease	Treatment dose	Efficacy	Adverse effects
Calugareanu et al.[3]	16 (9)	56	7/16	NA	5×↑↑↑	Conjunctivitis (2 patients)
					9×↑↑	Worsening of coeliac disease (1 patient)
					2×→	Eosinophilia (1 patient)
Napolitano et al.[11]	9 (5)	50.1	9/9	600 mg induction, 300 mg every 2 weeks	9×↑↑	None
Ferrucci et al.[4]	11 (5)	51	11/11	600 mg induction, 300 mg every 2 weeks	5×↑↑↑ 4×↑↑	Acute psoriasiform dermatitis (1 patient)
Rambhia et al.[12]	2 (2)	46.5	No	600 mg induction, 300 mg every 2 weeks	1×↑↑ 1×↑	Alopecia (1 patient)
Calugareanu et al.[13]	1 (1)	30	Yes	600 mg induction, 300 mg every 2 weeks	↑↑↑	None
Beck et al.[14]	3 (1)	61	NA	600 mg induction, 300 mg every 2 weeks	3×↑↑↑	Herpes labialis (1 patient)
Mollanazar et al.[15]	4 (3)	40's	2/4	600 mg induction, 300 mg every 2 weeks	4×↑↑↑	None
Almustafa et al.[16]	3 (1)	46	3/3	600 mg induction, 300 mg every 2 weeks	3×↑↑	None

(NA: not available, Overall effect; → none, ↑ mild, ↑↑ moderate, ↑↑↑ complete)

KEY MESSAGE

- Dupilumab may be an effective and well-tolerated option for treatment of chronic PN not controlled with other treatments.

REFERENCES

1. Tsianakas A, Zeidler C, Ständer S. Prurigo nodularis management. Curr Probl Dermatol 2016;5094-101.
2. Olesen CM, Holm JG, Nørreslet LB, Serup JV, Thomsen SF, Agner T. Treatment of atopic dermatitis with dupilumab : experience from a tertiary referral centre. J Eur Acad Dermatol Venereol. 2019;33:1562-8.
3. Calugareanu A, Jachiet M, Tauber M, Nosboum A, Aubin F, Misery L, et al. Effectiveness and safety of dupilumab for the treatment of prurigo nodularis in a French multicenter adult cohort of 16 patients. J Eur Acad Dermatology Venereol. 2020;34:e74-6.
4. Ferrucci S, Tavecchio S, Berti E, Angileri L. Dupilumab and prurigo nodularis-like phenotype in atopic dermatitis: our experience of efficacy. J Dermatolog Treat. 2019;1-2.
5. Wieser JK, Mercurio MG, Somers K. Resolution of treatment-refractory prurigo nodularis with dupilumab: A case series. Cureus 2020;12(6):e8737.

6. Romano C. Safety and effectiveness of dupilumab in prurigo nodularis. J Investig Allergol Clin Immunol. 2020; doi:10.18176/jiaci.0550.
7. Criado PR, Pincelli TP, Criado RFJ. Dupilumab as a useful treatment option for prurigo nodularis in an elderly patient with atopic diathesis. Int J Dermatol. 2020; doi:10.1111/ijd.14994.
8. Kovács B, Rose E, Kuznik N, Simanovich I, Zillikens D, Ludwig RJ, et al. Dupilumab for treatment-refractory prurigo nodularis. JDDG - J Ger Soc Dermatology. 2020;18:618-24.
9. Holm JG, Agner T, Sand C, Thomsen SF. Dupilumab for prurigo nodularis: Case series and review of the literature. Dermatol Ther. 2020;33(2):e13222.
10. Giura MT, Viola R, Fierro MT, Ribero S, Ortoncelli M. Efficacy of dupilumab in prurigo nodularis in elderly patient. Dermatol Ther 2020; 33(1):e13201:doi:10.1111/dth.13201.
11. Napolitano M, Fabbrocini G, Scalvenzi M, Nistico SP, Dastoli S, Patruno C. Effectiveness of dupilumab for the treatment of generalized prurigo nodularis phenotype of adult atopic dermatitis. Dermatitis. 2020; doi:10.1097/DER.0000000000000517.
12. Rambhia PH, Levitt JO. Recalcitrant prurigo nodularis treated successfully with dupilumab. JAAD Case Rep. 2019;5:471-3.
13. Calugareanu A, Jachiet M, Lepelletier C, Masson AD, Rybojad M, Bagot M, et al. Dramatic improvement of generalized prurigo nodularis with dupilumab. J Eur Acad Dermatology Venereol. 2019;33:e303-4.
14. Beck K, Yang E, Sekhon S, Bhutani T, Liao W. Dupilumab treatment for generalized prurigo nodularis. JAMA Dermatol. 2019;155:118-20.
15. Mollanazar N, Elgash M, Weaver L, Valdes-Rodriguez R, Hsu S. Reduced itch associated with dupilumab treatment in 4 patients with prurigo nodularis. JAMA Dermatol. 2019; 155:121-2.
16. Almustafa ZZ, Weller K, Autenrieth J, Maurer M, Metz M. Dupilumab in treatment of chronic prurigo: A case series and literature review. Acta Derm Venereol. 2019;99:905-6.

Index

Page numbers followed by *b* refer to box, *f* refer to figure, and *t* to table.

A

Abrocitinib 60
Achyranthes aspera 80
Acitretin 124
Allergens 4
  penetration of 55
Allergic contact dermatitis 20, 40, 41, 55, 63, 69, 70
  diagnosis of 40
Allergic diseases 16
Allium cepa 80
Allium sativum 80
Aloe vera 80
Antibiotics, systemic 98
Antifungals
  systemic 110
  topical 110
Antihistamine 106
Antineutrophil cytoplasmic antibody 94
Antinuclear antibody 94
Anxiety 15, 86
Arterial hypertension, systemic 11
Arthropod bites 120
Aspirin 89
Asthma 79
  childhood-onset 62
  personal history of 22
  severe 62
Atopic dermatitis 1, 3, 6, 8, 8*f*, 9, 10, 15, 19, 21, 22*b*, 25, 27, 29, 30, 33, 35, 36, 38, 40, 41, 48, 51-53, 55, 57, 60*t*, 62, 63, 65, 65*f*, 66, 66*f*, 67, 70, 74, 76-79, 86, 87, 117, 120, 124
  adult-onset 62, 63
  classic early onset 32
  erythrodermic early onset 32
  pathogenesis of 55
  refractory 29
    severe 72
  reliable estimation of 22
  severe 3, 27, 52, 65
    adult-onset 19
    refractory 72
Atopic disease 11, 22
Atopy 79
  family history of 22
  personal history of 22
Autoimmune blistering disease 119
Azadirachta indica 80, 81
Azathioprine 13, 17, 29, 53, 65, 74, 85, 124

B

Baricitinib 60
Bauhinia variegata 80
Benralizumab 108, 108*f*, 109, 109*f*, 109*t*, 110
Biliary cholangitis, primary 15
Bladder, metastatic transitional cell carcinoma of 15
Blepharitis 67
Blepharoconjunctivitis, recurrent herpetic 65*f*
Boric acid compresses 5
Brachioradial pruritus 15
Bullous pemphigoid 45
Burns 58

C

Calcineurin inhibitors, topical 29, 62
Calcitonin gene-related peptide 15
Carbamazepine 48
Cataracts, anterior subcapsular 22
Celiac disease 15, 119
Cheilitis 22
Chikungunya infections, 14
Cholesterol ointment 5
Chronic autoimmune cholestatic hepatitis 15
Chronic inflammatory
  disease 33
  disorder 6
Chronic obstructive pulmonary disease 20
Clostridium difficile 5
Collagen fibers 15
Colophony 40, 41
Complete blood count 59, 62
Conjunctivitis 21, 30, 67, 70
  allergic 22
  recurrent 22
Contact allergy 38
Contact dermatitis 41, 117
Contrail sign 123
Coronavirus disease 17
Corticosteroid
  systemic 65, 98
  topical 29, 62, 69
COVID-19 17
C-reactive protein 20, 59, 62, 114
Cross-reactive carbohydrate determinant 5
Cutaneous lesions, evolution of 12*f*
Cutaneous pruriginous recurrent lesions 98
Cutaneous T-cell lymphoma 15, 21, 63
Cyclosporine 17, 29, 35, 37, 53, 65, 74, 85, 106, 110

D

Dapsone, systemic 110
Darier's disease 67
Darier–White disease 58
Delgocitinib 60
Delta glider sign 123

Demodex-associated rosacea-like dermatitis 70
Dendritic cells 15
Dengue 14
Dennie–Morgan infraorbital fold 22
Depression 15, 86
Dermal fibrosis 12
Dermal perivascular lymphocytic infiltrate 85
Dermatitis 22, 33, 55, 69
 herpetiformis 117, 119, 120
Dermatology life quality index 25, 26, 29, 33, 52, 69, 72, 86, 126
Dermatome 15
Dermatosis, benign 77
Dermographism 113
 diagnosis of 112
Dermoscopic clues 114
Dermoscopic examination 122f
Dermoscopy 123
Diabetes mellitus 15, 20, 79
DiGeorge syndrome 48, 49
Doxycycline 96
Drug reaction with eosinophilia and systemic symptoms syndrome 48
Dry eye 67
Dry skin 10
Duhring–Brocq disease 119
Dupilumab 11, 16, 19, 25, 30, 33, 34, 53, 63, 65, 67, 71, 124, 127, 127t, 128
 therapy 14, 69
Dupilumab-induced face dermatitis 62
Dyslipidemia 89
Dystrophic epidermolysis bullosa 45

E

Eczema 104
 area and severity index 17, 26, 33, 52, 69, 86
 score 25, 32
 herpeticum 57, 58, 65, 67
 skin lesions of 58f
Electroencephalogram 48
Emollients 5
Encephalitis 59
Endothelial cells 15

Eosinophil 104
 cationic protein 15, 109t
Eosinophilia 22, 109t
Eosinophilic folliculitis 108
 pathogenesis of 110
Eosinophilic perifolliculitis 107
Epidermal keratinocytes 15
Epidermolysis bullosa
 pruriginosa 44, 45
 skin lesions 45f
Erythematous papules 95, 112, 113f, 114, 121f
Erythematous patches 39f
Erythematous-desquamative mild infiltrated plaques 12f
Erythrocyte sedimentation rate 20, 59, 72, 94
Erythroderma 34
Extensor eruptions 22
Extractable nuclear antibody 94
Extracutaneous nerves 15
Eye pruritus 67

F

Facial eruptions 22
Facial pallor 22
Fast recurrent dermatitis 41
Fever 59
Filaggrin 73
Fitzpatrick's skin 11
Flexural involvement, history of 22
Flexural lichenification 22
Food
 allergens 4t
 allergy 35–37
 intolerance 22
Foot dermatitis 22
Full blood count 114
Fungal skin infection 9
Fungal vellus hair 9f
Fungoides 32

G

Gabapentin 17, 124
Gamma benzene hexachloride 91
Generalized dry skin, history of 22
Generalized purpuric macules 89

Gilbert syndrome 57
Global Initiative for Asthma Guidelines 62
Gout 15
Gusacitinib 60

H

Hailey–Hailey disease 58
Hand dermatitis 22
 refractory 41
Hand eczema, worsening of 40
Hanifin and Rajka diagnostic criteria 22
Hay fever 22
Headache 70
Heart disease, ischemic 79
Hepatitis
 B 94
 chronic 15
 C 15, 94
Herpes infections 70
Herpes simplex viruses 58, 67
Histamine 15
HIV infection 15
Hodgkin lymphoma 15
Hospital anxiety and depression scale 86
Hydrochlorothiazide 89
Hypereosinophilia 107
Hypergranulosis 85
Hyperkeratosis 85
Hyperkeratotic epidermis 12
Hyperkeratotic plaques 39f, 40
Hyperpigmentation 96
Hypertension 79, 89
Hypopigmented polymorphous light eruption 77

I

Ichthyosis 22, 67
 vulgaris 58
Immediate skin test reaction 22
Immunoglobulin E 26, 29, 66, 85, 112, 114
 specific 5
Immunomodulators, topical 69
Impaired cell-mediated immunity 22
Incipient bullous pemphigoid 15
Inflammatory skin disease 127

Influenza 36
Injection site reactions 70
Intense xerosis 15
Intensive pruritus 117
Internal malignancies 15
International Alliance for
    Control of Scabies Criteria
    91
Iron-deficiency anemia 15
Irregular acanthosis 12
Itching 22, 38, 89
Itchy rash 124
Itchy red raised lesions 121
Itchy skin condition 22
Itchy small papules 104, 105*f*
Itchy urticarial lesions 93

J

Janus family protein kinases
    16
Janus kinase 27
    inhibitors 57, 60, 60*t*
Juvenile eosinophilic
    folliculitis 107, 110
    primary 110
    treatment of 110

K

Kang and Tian diagnostic
    criteria 22
Kaposi varicelliform eruption
    58
Keratitis 67
Keratoconus 22
Keratosis pilaris 22
Keto rash 96
Kidney
    failure, chronic 15
    function 48

L

Lactate dehydrogenase 26
Leukocytoclastic vasculitis 90*f*,
    91
Lichen planus 15
Lichenoid papules 45*f*
Liver
    diseases 15
    function tests 48
Localized prurigo nodularis 15
Loratadine 98

Low-potent topical
    corticosteroid 78
Lymphadenopathy 59
Lymphocytes 104
Lymphocytic infiltration 96

M

Macrolides 110
Malaise 59
Malassezia furfur-associated
    dermatitis 70
Manidipine 89
Mast cells 15
Measles 36
Merkel cells 15
Methotrexate 17, 29, 53, 65, 74
Microsporum canis 10
Minitriangle sign 123
Minocycline 96
Mometasone furoate 5
Monoclonal gammopathy 15
Monoclonal T-cell receptor 32
Montelukast 106
Multiple drug allergies 51
Multiple eosinophilic
    granulocytes 108*f*
Multiple organ involvement 59
Mumps 36
Mycophenolate 53
    mofetil 13, 17
Mycosis fungoides 21, 58, 63,
    67, 77

N

Nagashima disease 96
Nasal fluticasone 53
Nasopharyngitis 70
Nerve
    cutaneous 15
    growth factor 15
Neuropathic diseases 15
Neuropathic pruritus 15
Neutrophils 104
Nevus depigmentosus 77
Nipple eczema 22
Nodules 85
Non-Hodgkin's lymphoma 15
Noninfectious pruritic
    dermatosis 108
Numerical rating scale 33, 86
Numerous keratinocytes,
    necrosis of 96

O

Obstructive sleep apnea 20
Omalizumab 44, 46, 72, 74
Oral corticosteroids 62, 69
Oral dapsone 96
Oral fluconazole 9
Oral hydroxyzine 98
Oral immunosuppressants 69
Oral valacyclovir 66

P

Palmar hyperlinearity 22
Papules 98
Papulopustular dermatosis 107
Paradoxical erythema 71
Parakeratosis foci 12
Paraphenylenediamine 40, 41,
    41*f*
Patch test 29, 41, 56, 69, 85
    reactions 41*f*
Patchy scaling erythema 70*f*
Patient-oriented eczema
    measure 86
Pemphigus
    foliaceus 58
    vulgaris 67
Periorbital darkening 22
Photophobia 65
Photosensitivity reaction, drug-
    induced 63
Phototherapy 17
Physician global assessment
    33, 126
Pimecrolimus 52, 53
Pityriasis 77
    alba 22, 77
        lesions of 78
        pigmentary variant of 78
Polymerase chain reaction 59
Polymyositis 94
Popliteal fossa 22, 40
Positive patch test reactions,
    relevance of 40
Postherpetic neuralgia 15
Post-steroid hypopigmentation
    77
Potassium hydroxide 9*f*, 77
Prednisolone 52, 53, 124
Pregabalin 17
Prick test 29
Progressive itchy rash 8*f*
Progressive skin lesions 89

Prostaglandins 15
Pruriginous atopic eczema 14
Prurigo nodularis 11, 14, 15b, 16, 18, 85, 87, 124, 126, 127, 127t
 clinical grade for 15b
 diagnosis of 85
Prurigo pigmentosa 95, 96
 histopathological features of 95f
 rash of 94f
Pruritic bullous lesions 44
Pruritic dermatitis 22
Pruritic eruption 117
Pruritic papules 85
Pruritus 22, 69, 74, 83, 104, 108
Psoriasiform epidermal hyperplasia 85
Psoriasis 21, 63, 77
Psoriatic arthritis 60
Psychiatric disorders 15
Purpuric macules 89f
Pustular rash 65

R

Rabies 36
Randomized controlled trials 74
Rapid-eye-movement sleep 37
Rash 38, 94f
Renal transplantation 3
Retinoids 110
Rheumatoid arthritis 60
Rhinitis, allergic 14, 21, 52
Rubella 36
Ruxolitinib 60

S

Sarcoptes scabiei 90f, 100, 101, 114, 121, 123
Scabies 21, 63, 91, 102, 112, 116, 120
 incognito 99f, 102t
 diagnosis of 112, 115
 types of 115, 115t
Scabietic vasculitis 91
Scaly patches 39f
Scleroderma 94
Scoring atopic dermatitis 52, 62, 66, 69
 index 72
 scale 4
 score 35

Seborrhea 77
Septate hyphae 9f
Serpiginous burrow 114f
Severe eczematous dermatitis 19
Sézary disease 32
Sézary syndrome 58
Simvastatin 89
Skin
 biopsy 77, 90, 90f, 107
 celiac disease of 119
 eruptions 73f
 generalized dryness of 40
 infection 91
 inflammatory disease 73
 lesions 58f, 76f, 86f, 118f
 prick tests 52, 85
 swelling of 112
Spleen tyrosine kinase 60
Staphylococcus aureus 59
Stevens–Johnson syndrome 48
Stratum corneum 101
Sulfonamides 110
Sunset yellow dye, structure of 50f
Sweating 22
Systemic immunosuppressive therapies 61

T

Tacrolimus, topical 110
Tactile hallucinations 15
T-cell-driven complex inflammatory skin disease 74
Telmisartan 89
Tetracycline 96, 110
Thalidomide 17, 124
Therapy-resistant dermatitis 41
Thermal burns 67
Thymic stromal lymphopoietin 59
Thyroid disease 15
Tinea
 corporis 77
 incognito 9
 infection 9
 versicolor 77
Tofacitinib 60
Total prostatic-specific antigen 11

Toxocara canis 11
Trichophyton mentagrophytes 9
Tuberous sclerosis, ash leaf macules of 77
Tyrosine kinase 60

U

Ulcerative colitis 60
Ultraviolet light
 A 124, 126
 B 124, 126
United Kingdom Working Party's Diagnostic Criteria 22
Upadacitinib 60
Urticaria 104
 chronic spontaneous 46
Urticarial vasculitis 93

V

Varicella-herpes zoster virus 60
Vasculitis, cutaneous 91
Viremia 59
Visual analog sleep 86
Visual analogue scale 14, 25, 124, 126
Vitiligo 77

W

White blood cell 62
White dermographism 22
Wiskott–Aldrich syndrome 67
Wood's lamp 77

X

Xerosis 22, 39f

Y

Yellow fever 36
 vaccine 36

Z

Zika virus 14